D1569040

THE

Mindfulness

DIET

Dr. Patrizia Collard
& Helen Stephenson

An Hachette UK Company
www.hachette.co.uk

First published in Great Britain in 2015 by
Gaia Books, a division of Octopus Publishing Group Ltd
Endeavour House
189 Shaftesbury Avenue
London WC2H 8JY
www.octopusbooks.co.uk
www.octopusbooksusa.com

Distributed in the US by Hachette Book Group
1290 Avenue of the Americas
4th and 5th Floors
New York, NY 10020

Distributed in Canada by Canadian Manda Group
664 Annette Street,
Toronto, Ontario, Canada M6S 2C8

ISBN 978 0 60063 051 7

Printed and bound by CPI Group (UK) Ltd, Croydon, CR0 4YY
10 9 8 7 6 5 4 3 2 1

Commissioning Editor Liz Dean
Designer Jeremy TIlston
Production Controller Sarah Kramer

Any information given in this book is not intended to be taken as a replacement for medical
advice. Any person with a condition requiring medical attention should consult a qualified
practitioner or therapist.

Calorie counts for recipes do not include serving suggestions.

Contents

Introduction

How often do we think about food, or the effect food has on our body? We are living in a culture that is obsessed with the young, the good-looking, and the slim. Although we know that people in the public eye often have personal trainers, and some have eating disorders and possibly drug issues, we still feel inadequate in comparison. We are aware that a professional photoshoot takes ages and the pictures that are finally published have been manipulated and retouched, but nevertheless we compare ourselves to the models shown in them. Most of us, to a greater or lesser degree, are unhappy with the way we look and whether we relate that to our eating habits or not, we think about food many times during the day. Here are some of the thoughts that may occur to you. Read them and add your own.

- What do I want to eat now?
- What did I eat yesterday, the day before?
- What will I eat tomorrow?
- Why did I eat this? I wish I hadn't eaten it.
- I will never eat carbohydrates/sugar/meat from now on.
- What should I eat?
- What shouldn't I eat?
- I am happy/unhappy with the way I look, or the way my body looks.

Research figures suggest that the number of thoughts people have about food alone can be anything up to 200 per day. The number might be a great deal higher, if thoughts about body image are added to that. Food tops the stakes in the overall thought-count. We have received enough public education to know what we need to eat to be healthy. We know what food we should eat in small quantities to avoid obesity and all the health issues that go with it, such as hypertension and heart disease. And still we face the same image in the mirror—nothing changes.

Most days we can accept how we look, but some days, even if the sun is shining brightly, our mind can shift to a state in which we see the world through the eyes of fat and slim. This is what we may start thinking when we enter that frame of mind:

- I am going on vacation soon; can I still wear the bikini from last year?

- I should go for some exercise, then I can have that delicious Italian homemade ice cream.
- Should I skip the evening meal to lose a tiny weeny bit of weight around the waist?
- Should I book a personal trainer to get in shape for the vacation?

When we are in "battle mode," we may forget the many gifts that have been bestowed upon us—a healthy body, good skin, full hair, and a sharp and curious brain. Mindfulness and compassion can help you to accept yourself at a deeper level and to achieve a much more joyful and wholesome relationship with food.

Definition of mindfulness

Mindfulness lies at the core of Buddhist meditative practices but it is universal. It can be described as a way of being, a way of seeing, and a way of connecting to your senses.

> *"The present is the only time that any of us have to be alive, to know anything, to perceive, to learn, to act, to change, to heal."*
> **JON KABAT-ZINN**

Staying in touch with the present in a mindful way from one moment to the next may lead to you experiencing life differently. You may become a little less stuck in your ways, perceiving more options and finding more strength, more balance, more understanding, and confidence. The practice of mindfulness can diffuse our negativity, aggression, and unstable emotions.

Mindfulness has also been described as "bare attention." That term was coined by German-born Buddhist monk N Thera, one of the great figures of 20th-century Buddhism. It is called "bare" because it attends just to the bare facts of perception as presented, either through the five senses or through the mind, without reacting to them or judging them. We behave rather like an outside observer, perceiving what is happening to us, accepting and allowing it. The thoughts or feelings we observe are not us, they are just something that is happening to us.

History of mindfulness

The origins of mindfulness go back to the Suthras of 2500 BCE, and it has connections to Taoist and Yogic philosophy. The first text of importance in the 20th century is *The Miracle of Mindfulness* by the Vietnamese monk Thich Nhat Hanh. This was originally written as a letter from exile in France to one of the brothers who had remained in Vietnam.

The school that Hanh had founded in the 1960s was intended to help rebuild bombed villages, teach children, and set up medical stations for both sides engaged in the conflict. The letter's intention was to support the brothers back home, encouraging them to continue to work in a spirit of love and understanding. Hanh simply wished to remind them of the essential discipline of mindfulness, even in the midst of very difficult circumstances.

At the time Hanh was writing the letter in Paris, several supporters from different countries were attending the Vietnamese Buddhist Peace Delegation. So it was quite natural to think of people in other countries who might also benefit from reading this letter. Hanh suggested the translator, an American volunteer, should translate it slowly and steadily, in order to maintain mindfulness. Thus only two pages a day were translated. Hanh encouraged the translator to be aware of the feel of the pen and paper, to be aware of the position of his body, and to be aware of his breath in order to maintain the essence of mindfulness while doing this task. When the translation was completed, it was typed and a hundred copies were printed on a tiny offset machine squeezed into the delegation's bathroom. Since then the little book has traveled far.

It has been translated into many other languages and distributed on every continent in the world. Prisoners, refugees, healthcare workers, psychotherapists, educators, and artists are among those whose life and work has been touched by *The Miracle of Mindfulness*. Denied permission to return to Vietnam, Thich Nhat Hanh spends most of the year living in Plum Village, a community he helped found in France. He says of himself: "I am eighty-seven years young." Plum Village is open to visitors from around the world who wish to spend a mindfulness retreat there. The proceeds from the fruit of hundreds of plum trees are used to assist hungry children in Vietnam.

In the late 1970s, Jon Kabat-Zinn (Ph.D) started to apply mindfulness techniques to treating patients with chronic pain at Massachusetts Medical School. Due to the successful outcome of the initial patient groups treated with this approach, he started to develop his now world famous mindfulness-based stress reduction (MBSR) program. In 1991 the first book describing the program of the stress-reduction clinic at

Massachusetts Medical Center, entitled *Full Catastrophe Living*, was published and over half a million copies have been sold worldwide. Eventually, in 1989, at the World Congress of Cognitive Therapy held in Oxford, British psychologists and psychotherapists, searching for new treatment models for recurring depression, were introduced to mindfulness approaches. Mindfulness-based cognitive therapy for depression was the result of their studies and was first published in 2002.

Mindfulness-based cognitive therapy and relapse

Research estimates that around 20 percent of the population in Western countries will suffer an episode of clinical depression at least once in their lifetime. However, up until the 1990s, CBT (cognitive behavioral therapy) research did not explore the fact that patients who have had more than one or two episodes of depression are susceptible to becoming depressed again and again. Very little hard data focused on this phenomenon of "relapse" until researchers began to look for a more cost- and time-effective intervention to deal with it. Regular CBT would be used for acute depression and the "new approach" of MBSR would hopefully cater for relapse prevention.

John Teasdale (Ph.D) and others discovered that even minor increases in sadness could reactivate "depressive thinking neuro-pathways" in formerly depressed client groups. Cognitive behavioral psychotherapy had often been used to deactivate negative thinking but some remnants tended to stay behind, and these could not be "deleted" from the "hard disk" of the patient's mind. Each new episode of depression hardwires these depressive thought patterns more and more. Hence relapse tends to become more and more probable the more often a person has experienced clinical depression.

The fusion of mindfulness-based stress reduction (MBSR) and mindfulness-based cognitive therapy (MBCT)

Mindfulness-based cognitive therapy is an integration of mindfulness-based stress reduction with cognitive behavioral therapy. In conventional CBT, the focus is on changing unhelpful beliefs. In MBCT, the focus is rather on methodical training to be more aware, moment by moment, of physical sensations and of thoughts and feelings as mental events. Research on MBCT shows that it can halve the relapse rate in recovered patients who have had three or more episodes of depression. Other targeted versions of MBCT have now been developed, including MBCT for chronic-fatigue syndrome, for oncology patients, in schools, for anxiety disorders, and in the treatment of trauma, to mention just a few. Mindfulness-based eating interventions are being developed as we speak.

How MBCT works
- Identify your cognitive "distortions"—conscious awareness.
- Identify the fact that the imagined "threat" is only a thought.
- Sit with what "is"—I am okay, even now.
- Appraise your internal resources—"I can."

What is mindful eating?

This is not yet another diet book! We are confident that to deal with food, weight, and health issues we have to deal with the entire person, or as the founder of mindfulness-based stress reduction, Jon Kabat-Zinn, said in his first book, we have to deal with the "full catastrophe of living."

By buying *The Mindfulness Diet*, you have taken an important step away from the so-called experts and food fads toward your inner wisdom. This book is meant to help you trust yourself again. You are the expert, so make your own decisions. Nobody can make them for you. Nobody can live your life for you, shower for you, have sex for you, or eat for you.

By bringing mindfulness into your life, more specifically into your eating life, you will learn to stop, to tune in, and to listen. You will become interested in what is really important to you. Through the various practices in this book, you make time and pay attention to what is going on in your life right now. You will come to understand how your thoughts and feelings, if unnoticed, can pull you away from the present moment, and make you go for the candy bar to avoid the discomfort of feeling upset or lonely.

When we pay attention to our food intake, we have to face our true longings and explore what we really want. Could it be that we want to be in touch with our bodies and our senses? Or do we also want to be in touch with our true self, and would we like to live an authentic life of self-care and other-care.

By not being mindful with our "true" hunger, we tend to eat more, when having less could be what is needed. By becoming mindful we develop understanding, and in this process we become more forgiving and kinder to ourselves. Just by reading this book you can start to replace hating your body with appreciating your inner wisdom. You can release yourself from the grip of shame and anger and replace it with understanding. You will become less obsessed about food and how you look and more attuned to the appreciation of being alive.

How to use this book

The chapters in this book explore different influences and factors that affect the way we eat mindfully. At the end of each chapter you'll find a handful of recipes that we encourage you to prepare and eat mindfully. The first example is a more detailed guided practice. After that you'll find "Awareness Points" at the end of each recipe with tips for things to look out for and appreciate.

The recipes are particularly relevant for the topics explored in each chapter, but feel free to pick and choose recipes from any place in the book. You'll find a list of recipes on page 152–53.

There is a food journal template on page 103 where you can record your eating habits and a one-month mindful eating plan at the end of the book.

As you progress, apply the lessons you have learned and think of your own awareness points for the recipes you cook and meals you eat.

Reading this book, and practicing the exercises, will help you to:

• reconnect with your body and its senses
• retrain yourself to enjoy your food without guilt and shame

- feel full and eat less as you learn to feel truly nourished
- break free from destructive eating habits
- become aware of the feelings and thoughts that keep your unhelpful eating patterns in place
- reconnect with your own inner wisdom
- live life with zest and creativity
- free yourself from negative thinking and develop compassion and kindness.

Factors that influence our eating habits

- **The genetic code**
  "I have big bones." It is obvious that some people have a larger frame than others, but holding onto the idea that our weight is dictated solely by genetics assumes that change is impossible. Mindful eating invites us to accept the fact that we cannot change the basic frame of our body, but that we can still find our own ideal weight, together with a healthy sense of appreciation and respect for our body.

- **Reward and punishment**
  There are countless times when we have eaten something unhealthy (and delicious) because "we are worth it"; and times when we have felt obliged to eat something that we don't like. We may assume it's normal to live with this inner struggle of "I must" and "I mustn't." But the mind that says "I must not ..." and the mind that says "I must ..." are one and the same. Instead of engaging in this inner conflict, we can step back and clearly see the dynamics at play. By becoming a witness to the feelings, a space is created around them and we are no longer a hostage to them, acting from a place of confusion and frustration.

- **The teenage years**
  Being a teenager marks the beginning of a very important period in our life. It is a time of constant changes in the body and a time when we become self-conscious about our size and eating habits. During this period, views are formed about how we see ourselves and how others see us. You might still be holding onto a painful story about your teenage years. But now it is important to acknowledge that whatever it was happened in the past. By accepting that, you allow yourself to move on. Mindfulness enables us to let go of those stories and feelings, and to replace them with what is needed now.

- **Emotions**

  Very few people in the West eat out of hunger alone. Most of us eat from a place of emotion. We often do things, such as eating chocolate while watching TV, without being conscious of the thoughts and feelings that drive the behavior. We live and eat on autopilot, reacting to signals from the brain or cravings from the mind. Mindfulness is about having the awareness to see the formation of the emotion, to see its origins and, with practice, even to see the very first thought that started it all.

- **Lack of exercise**

  We live in a sedentary world. Products are consistently delivered, enabling us to be less active. The voices of the medical profession are drowned out by the noises that encourage us to do less and eat more. Research suggests that walking every day for at least 15 minutes is an important factor in improving health. Exercise is one of our best supports in achieving our ideal weight, size, and shape.

- **Addictions**

  We experience the strength of addiction when we feel forced to eat the chocolate, when we are desperate to open that package and when we experience a feeling of no choice, of inevitability.

  The other factor involved in addiction is big business. The food industry exists to sell food, and making us go back for more is what the product is designed to do. By recognizing this fact, we are released from feelings of failure and weakness, and with mindfulness we will be able to break this cycle.

- **Alcohol**

  Alcohol creates a mind that is open to suggestion and more willing to throw away caution, and is responsible for a lot of bad food choices. We may go to the bar and stop for a burger, or stay in and relax on the couch with a drink and a bag of potato chips. Alcohol *really* has the potential to derail any attempts to change your shape or weight. It is one of the most concentrated sources of calories with little nutritional value. If you want to become more mindful around food, moderating alcohol consumption is a must.

- **Social pressure**

  Eating with others is wonderful but we may make choices that we would never make if we were eating alone, and we eat with only a fraction of the awareness that we might usually feel. Knowing this helps you to approach those situations calmly, and by being clear about the choices you have, you can act in accordance with your values and wishes. If you decide to go for that second delicious dessert, you will be doing it consciously, and savoring it, and you won't feel guilty afterward, because you were fully aware of the consequences.

- **Laziness**
  Even the most efficient and focused person will occasionally think, "I can't be bothered to cook tonight." The feeling of tiredness or laziness is not the problem, but how we relate to it, because the food choices that we make in this moment will have an impact on our body.

  This is where mindfulness comes into play: seeing the feeling and not identifying with it, and so separating it from yourself, will help you to respond with calm. Then you will be more likely to make a healthy choice, instead of simply following the usual habitual patterns.

- **Sleep**
  Sleep can impact on weight and eating habits. When people are sleeping less, the accumulation of body fat appears to increase—by up to 32 percent. According to one study, in less than two weeks of having their sleep disturbed on a nightly basis, participants increased their weight by an average of 3 lb.

  Also, when people suffer from daytime sleepiness, they are far more likely to crave high-sugar foodstuff. Mindfulness in general might help us to sleep better and to make the positive choices that will help us to avoid the weight gain.

- **Stress**
  During stress, the mind is on reaction mode as opposed to responding mode. The stress hormone cortisol interferes with the digestion of food, can lead to food cravings, and plays a significant part in people putting on weight. It speeds up the accumulation of fat around the waistline, while at the same time breaking down highly prized lean muscle.

  Mindfulness practices have been shown to trigger the "relaxation response," a series of physical reactions that are associated with a greater feeling of comfort and ease. The body goes into a positive cycle of wellbeing as high blood pressure decreases, breathing slows down, and muscle tension releases. The mind recognizes that the body is relaxing and therefore relaxes itself, which in turn reinforces and further promotes relaxation in the body. And so the positive loop continues, with body and mind winding down and easing up.

Mindful eating as a way of life— 10 tips

1. Listen to your body

Before you pile a mountain of food on your plate or break open a family-sized bag of chips, take a moment to listen to your physical needs. Are you hungry? If you are, how hungry are you? Serve up just enough food to satisfy the hunger of the body, rather than trying to quench the limitless desire of the mind. You'll be much less likely to go back for more than if you simply had the package of chips sitting on your lap.

2. Use smaller serving plates and bowls

Studies have shown that our satisfaction is tied in to "relative" portion sizes. So, if we have a very small plate that is piled high with food, we will feel much more satisfied than if we have a large plate with a small amount of food—even if the large serving on the small plate contains less! Some new crockery could be the best investment you ever made.

3. Be flexible when eating out

Restaurant menus are generally written in a way that encourages you to eat as much as possible (and why wouldn't they be?) but you don't have to play that game. There is no obligation to have an appetizer, entrée, and dessert. Why not have appetizers instead of an entrée? Why not have tea or coffee instead of a dessert for a change? Oh, and don't be afraid to ask for excess food to be put in a doggy-bag.

4. Serve up at source

When serving food at home, try to plate it up by the oven or stove, rather than at the table. If the excess is on the table in front of you while you are eating, then that's where your mind is likely to be. Studies have shown that you are likely to eat faster with the excess in front of you. Presumably this is prompted by some survival instinct from the past, when we weren't sure where the next meal was coming from.

5. When you eat, just eat

Portion sizes are intimately related to "how" we eat. For example, if you sit down at a table with a large box of chocolates and no distractions, you are unlikely to polish off the entire box. This is partly because you would be more aware of hunger levels, but also because you would probably feel greedy, embarrassed, or ashamed. But when you're watching TV or involved in another activity, this awareness can be drowned out.

6. Learn what a portion size is

If you want to become more mindful of portion sizes, and possibly even to follow the recommended quantities with certain foods, it can be really useful to know and understand what portion sizes are (quite different from "serving sizes," incidentally, which can be frighteningly large). As a general rule, a "cup" is about the size of a large tennis ball, 3¼ oz of meat is about the size of a deck of cards, and 1¼ oz cheese is about the size of a domino. This may help you to avoid having to weigh everything.

7. Think little and often

Many people overeat at meals because they are worried they might feel hungry later on. The body doesn't really work like this and all overeating tends to do is increase the dramatic swings in blood-sugar levels that will, in all likelihood, have you reaching for the cookie tin. Try to maintain a stable blood-sugar level and moderate level of satiety by eating small meals throughout the day, rather than just a couple of ridiculously large meals.

8. Have a salad as an appetizer

We often dive into large portions of rich and color-dense foods simply because we're hungry. The truth is, in these situations, we're often so hungry that we'd eat just about anything. So be smart and eat some raw vegetables or salad to burn off that extreme hunger before the meal itself. That way you will not feel the same need to overindulge in richer-tasting foods.

9. Have a glass of water before eating

The sensation of thirst is often confused with the feeling of hunger, so that whenever we feel thirsty, we tend to reach out for a snack, or, if about to serve up a meal, we're likely to put more food on the plate. To ensure that you are listening to the right signals, sip a good-size glass of water in the 10–15 minutes leading up to a meal. This way you can be sure that you are serving up only what the body actually needs.

10. Shop smart

Bulk-buying foods can often enable you to pick up some great bargains, but you know your own mind. If you are unable or unwilling to break those down into smaller portion sizes when you get home, then consider the possibility of buying smaller versions. While you may not get the same value for money, take a moment to think of the cost (financial, physical, mental, and emotional) of overeating large portions of food.

Frequently used practices

Once we start to engage in a friendly relationship with the body, the first foundation of mindfulness, our life becomes lighter and more joyful, easy and relaxed. There is no need to fight our body or treat it as an enemy— better to start with a feeling of wonder that you have this body, and that it sustains you day and night. When you are able to accept the body, to respect and love it, you will not only become grateful to be in this body but you will become grateful for all existence.

The body scan

The key objective in doing the body scan is to enhance awareness of physiological sensations and to train your mind to stay focused over a longer than usual period of time on a particular task in the now. Lie down on a mat or bed, or sit upright on a chair, and focus for a while on the movement of the breath before directing attention to each region of the body and observing what happens when doing this. Each body scan is a new beginning, a new "NOW."

Practice for around 40 minutes six times per week, with no expectation or judgment of a particular outcome. Let go of ideas such as success, failure, and relaxation, and bring an open mind, curiosity, and a sense of adventure to the practice.

The body scan works on many levels. Firstly, it helps you to realize that you have a body; then, that the body is not an idea or statement, but a felt experience. You know that you have a body because you are aware of its sensations. Also, the body scan is a symbolic way of saying "you are important," because you are turning your attention to yourself. Remember, it is okay to spend time with yourself.

The body scan consists of three steps:

- Intentionally moving the attention to a selected area.
- Holding the awareness there and experiencing the sensations.
- Moving on.

The body scan will help you to engage in a friendly relationship with your physical home. You will become more independent of other people's views, of how you should be and what you should look like. Eventually, you will arrive back home, finding the original happiness of being in this body.

By regularly practicing the body scan you will make some good discoveries:

- Paying attention is a good practice. Most of us find it relatively easy to focus on our bodies. By paying attention to your body, you make it "happy" as you trigger its relaxation response.
- It helps you to reconnect with your body and understand its language.
- It is a good way to be nice to yourself. Remember you are your own best friend. By turning to your body, you are nourishing yourself. You are appreciating it as it is right now, acknowledging that the body serves us day in day out and sustains us in the best possible way. It is our home!

When you start to practice body scan, do it in the morning. Normally, when we wake up our minds are not yet busy, so it is easier to focus. Of course, you should choose the time that is best for you—some of us are larks and others are owls. Here is a brief description of the actual exercise:

- Take a few moments to get in touch with the movement of your breath and the sensations in your body. Remind yourself of the intention of this practice. Its aim is not to feel any different, relaxed, or calm—this may happen or it may not. Instead, the intention of the practice is, as best you can, to bring awareness to any sensations you detect as you focus your attention on each part of the body in turn.

- Now bring the focus of your awareness down the left leg, into the left foot. Focus on each of the toes of the left foot in turn, bringing a gentle curiosity to investigating the quality of sensations you find. When you are ready, on an in-breath, feel or imagine the breath entering the lungs, and then passing down into the abdomen, into the left leg, the left foot, and out to the toes of the left foot. Then, on the out-breath, feel or imagine the breath coming all the way back up, out of the foot, into the leg up through the abdomen, chest, and out through the nose. Just practice this "breathing into" as best you can, approaching it playfully.

- Next allow your awareness to expand into the rest of the foot, then to the ankle, the top of the foot, and right into the bones and joints. Move your awareness to the lower left leg—the calf, shin, and knee in turn.

- Continue to bring awareness, and a gentle curiosity, to the physical sensations in each part of the rest of the body in turn—to the upper left leg, the right toes, right foot, right leg, pelvic area, back, abdomen, chest, fingers, hands, arms, shoulder, neck, head, and face. In each area, as best as you can, bring the same detailed level of awareness and gentle curiosity to the bodily sensations present. As you leave each major area, breathe into it on the in-breath, and let go of that region on the out-breath.

- When you become aware of tension, or other intense sensations, in a particular part of the body, you can breathe into that region, using the in-breath gently to bring awareness right into the tension, and, as best as you can, have a sense of letting go, or releasing, on the out-breath.

- The mind will wander away from the breath and the body from time to time. That is entirely normal. It is what minds do. When you notice it, acknowledge it, noticing where the mind has gone off to, and then gently return your attention to the body scan.

- After scanninh the whole body in this way, spend a few minutes being aware of the body as a whole, and of the breath flowing freely in and out.

Breath–body–thoughts exercise

Our minds sometimes create their own interpretation of events, and this affects our reaction to them. Facts + self-deprecating thoughts = depressive interpretation of events (internal propaganda). Once a negative interpretation stream is started, contrary information is ignored and consistent information is noticed. Therapists used to think that these thoughts were caused by depression. Cognitive therapy teaches the opposite. Negative interpretation causes reduced self-esteem, increased guilt, interrupted concentration, and undermined social interaction, plus, possibly, biological effects (stress-response).

- Catch negative thoughts and treat them as hypothesis, not fact. Then seek ways to disprove the hypothesis (reality testing). In this way, we learn to recognize thoughts as thoughts and not as facts.
- Allow thoughts to enter, see how they make you feel/how you interpret them, and then bring your thoughts back to neutrality. Awareness!
- Take a few moments now to become aware of the thoughts that are arising in your mind. Imagine yourself sitting in a movie theater, watching an empty screen, just waiting for thoughts to come. When they come, can you see what exactly they are and what happens to them? Some of them will vanish as you become aware of them.

- Focus on specific body reactions and the feelings arising from negative thoughts, such as tension or anger. Observe and stand next to emotion, but do not be dragged down by it.

Everyday informal practices
Here are some examples of daily mindful activities to try.

- Go for a walk. Experience the miracle of moving, perhaps on your daily commute to work. Take in the area where you walk, keeping your eyes open and looking straight ahead of you and not down.
- When you brush your teeth, notice the sensations of the brush on each tooth. Are you thinking about the day or night ahead of you? Notice this and bring your attention back to brushing your teeth.
- In the shower, instead of writing lists in your head or planning a speech for the lunchtime meeting, really feel the water touching your body and be aware of its temperature. Smell the soap or shower gel, notice what it feels like on your skin, and feel your muscles relaxing. Then feel gratitude for the luxury of having water just for washing.
- When you hear a sound, any sound—a phone ringing, a passing car, an airplane above, a bird singing, a dog barking—kindly remember to embrace this moment and engage for a few minutes in mindful breathing and listening.

Four ways to free yourself from the tyranny of time

The first way is to remember that time is a convention but has no absolute meaning. Einstein is supposed to have said, "If you're sitting on a hot stove, a minute can seem like an hour, but if you're doing something pleasurable, an hour can seem like a minute."

The second way is to live more in the present rather than worrying about the past or the future, which usually produces anxiety and dissatisfaction. As one well-known saying has it: "the past is history, the future is unknown, the now is a gift—'the present'." Practically speaking, that means when you eat, concentrate on eating; and when you wash the dishes, really focus on the task. The essence of mindfulness in daily life is to make every moment you have your own. Even if you have to rush, rush mindfully.

The third way is to take some time off every day just to be (don't forget, we are human *beings*). In other words, have a formal mindfulness meditation time. It is rather like brushing your teeth—not a luxury but something we need to do every day that will also strengthen and support us in time to come. Make the commitment to practice nondoing, being nonjudgmental and residing in stillness.

The fourth way is to simplify your life in certain aspects. Examples clients have shared are not feeling they have to read the newspaper or watch the news every day, or clean certain areas of the house every day. You needn't become a slave to your habits.

- Time is relative.
- Live now.
- Just be.
- Simplify.

A first exercise in mindful eating —the raisin practice

Now is a good time to introduce you to our first practice, bearing in mind what you have read so far—a mindful-eating practice also called the raisin experience. It was devised by Jon Kabat-Zinn as a way to demonstrate that consciously turning your attention to what you are engaged with at the moment when it is happening enriches and deepens your daily life. Examples could be driving a car, eating a meal, holding your cell phone in your hand, drinking a cup of coffee.

In the raisin exercise, Jon invites you to eat one raisin mindfully— slowly and with awareness of all your senses. Participants often comment on the eye-opening effect this practice can have in relation to their eating patterns. Typical comments are:

- I noticed that no one raisin looks the same as another, in color, shape, or ridging.
- I noticed how much more satisfaction I got out of eating one raisin mindfully compared to my normal habit of eating them a handful at a time.
- I had a much more pleasurable experience, because the practice of mindfully eating the raisin gave me a heightened sense of its taste, color, and texture.
- I noticed how often I eat mindlessly, because my mind is all over the

place rather than focusing on the food in front of me. I mull over things that have recently happened, plan what to do after having eaten, or lose myself in all kinds of thoughts and fantasies.

- I was surprised how it brought back memories from my childhood with my family, as if it was yesterday.
- I was surprised how my sense of time changed. Normally, I am easily bored, but I was so absorbed in the practice that I didn't notice the time at all.

Before we start, let me tell you a story to illustrate the benefits that mindfulness can bring to your eating experience. To celebrate the successful completion of a business deal, and to honor a Western business partner, George was invited to eat one of Japan's most expensive and sought-after delicacies—a poisonous fish, prepared by a specially trained cook. While eating it, George marveled at this delicacy—the taste, the softness of the flesh, the subtlety of the aromas. Soon after he had finished his meal, the manager approached their table and profusely apologized. Due to a mistake in the kitchen, they had been served ordinary fish.

This shows two things—that perception influences taste and that heightened awareness can provide us with a richer and more satisfying eating experience.

Now let's start the practice.

BEFOREHAND

- All food is acceptable, as long as it is eaten mindfully, but it's better to avoid fast food until you understand the technique of eating mindfully.
- Try to avoid all possible distractions for the time of the practice, such as cell phones, tablets, TV, reading the newspaper, or even engaging in especially confrontational conversations.
- Sit and ground yourself by feeling your feet on the floor, your buttocks on the seat. Feel your entire posture. Do you feel tight or loose, collapsed or upright, tired or agitated, calm and collected or frazzled and all over the place? (There are more details on body awareness in Chapter 2 "The intelligent body." Read it if you want to.)
- Connect with your breathing. (Chapter 4 "No breath, no life" will deepen your understanding. Read it if you feel like it.)
- Ask yourself if you are hungry or just fancy a bite to eat.
- Are your thoughts/emotions encouraging you to eat something now? (See Chapter 4 "No breath, no life.")
- Are any of your senses, such as smell or sight, triggering your wish to eat?

PRACTICE

- Now *look* at what's on your plate and imagine that you are seeing it for the first time ever. You could imagine that you are coming from another part of this world, or even from another planet, or you are a small child. This may feel a bit ridiculous, but it is helpful if, for this moment, you try to perceive the items on your plate as if you have never seen them before.

- *Look* at the colors, the different textures, the forms, and the size. Do you see any patterns? If you hold an item of food, either with cutlery or your hands, and turn it around, does it look different from different angles? Is the light reflected differently, showing you light and darker areas? Are there details you didn't notice before?

- If you can *touch* it (raw food, bread, fruits, vegetables, snacks) what do you feel? Is it hard, soft, rough, smooth, wet, dry, sticky, hot, cool, heavy, light? Does it feel the same all over, or are there differences between different parts of it? Are you aware which hand is touching it? How do you hold the food? Gently or with tight pressure? Did you notice that your body knows how to pick up food and hold it, without you interfering?

- *Smell* it by moving it to your nose. Does it smell sweet, sour, bitter, salty, or kind of meaty? Is the smell strong or subtle, or overpowering? Have any memories, associations, or images occurred during this part of the practice? Have you already now decided if you want to eat what's on your plate or not? (More about the conditioning of our food preferences in Chapter 1 "The power of our senses.") Could you be encouraged to continue, even if you have decided that you might not like what's on your plate?

- When you are ready, and when you are willing to do so, put the food into your mouth. You can even place it on your lips to see how that feels. Did you notice the movement of the joints of your hand and arm, and the coordination necessary to bring the food to your mouth? But please, don't chew it yet. Once more feel its texture, weight, and taste, and experience how your tongue is moving it. Has the smell intensified? Is the texture changing? What about the *taste*?

- After moving it around with your tongue, and when you are ready, start to *chew* it. Does it make a sound? Do you feel embarrassed or disappointed, or do you like it? Does the chewing change the food's texture, taste, and moisture? Don't count your bites, let the body chew and let the body decide when to swallow. Does it go down in one big gulp or do you need to swallow several times? Can you feel it going down? How far can you feel it going down? At the back of your throat, reaching the stomach? Who made the decision to swallow? Your body or you?

- How do you feel now? Was that enough or do you want more? Do you feel full or still empty? Do you want to go for another bite? Are you sad that the food has gone?

- Thirty minutes to an hour after the meal, ask yourself: "How do I feel now?" Are you still hungry or are you satisfied? Are you very full, heavy or light, tired or energized? Knowing this could help you to make better choices next time around.

1 The power of our senses

I see it. I nearly forgot it was there. But there it is, on the shelf, not yet opened. I like it, I want it, I love it. My favorite spread—almond butter. This happens within seconds and I feel powerless. I must have it, I can't wait, I can even eat it with a spoon, no bread is needed.

You will have a different favorite food, but imagine that you know this feeling. So it might be worth having a closer look at what happens when our senses are triggered and how they can influence what we do and do not eat. All five senses are involved in wanting food, and enjoying it—taste, smell, sight, sound, and touch. They work together to give us a complete sensory experience, enabling us to savor our food (hmmm). It is the pleasure of this experience that we want to remember and repeat when we say that we liked and enjoyed the food.

Food choices and preferences

Many of our food preferences are learned and this learning begins before birth. Tests have shown that what women eat during pregnancy is easily detectable in their amniotic fluid, and the fetus develops a taste for these familiar flavors. Human beings are born to love sweetness. We love it in the womb. Fetuses aged between 15 and 16 weeks swallowed more amniotic fluid when it was sweet and less when it was bitter. The younger we are, the easier it is to mold the neural pathways. Chances are, if your mother liked garlic, you are going to like it, too.

But don't despair if your mother loved junk food and you think that now you are prone to eat and love only that. Other factors influence our food choices as we grow up, such as the power of advertising, peer pressure, and cultural influences.

Remember, mindful eating is about enjoying your food. Anything that takes your focus away makes it less likely that you will have the full experience of knowing what you are eating. When on autopilot, you might overeat without knowing it or consume food that is hardly nourishing.

Getting Started—
A Sensory Recipe Experience

Guided Practice: Thai Veg Salad

Mindful eating can be a strange first-time experience. You may want to try it out on your own at first. Find a time and place where you won't be interrupted by noise or work or the demands of other people. Make your kitchen into a peaceful, mindful space as far you can, and sit down to eat somewhere comfortable. You may not notice everything at first—as with all mindfulness practices, be kind to yourself, and if the mind wanders, simply guide it back to the meal at hand.

The first recipe here is simple and will take just 10 minutes to cook plus cooling time. It is full of bright and colorful ingredients to awaken the sense of sight, a wide variety of textures to explore, aromatic herbs and, most importantly, it has a fantastic, fresh taste. Take time to display and garnish the food so it looks appetizing—a dish you are proud of having prepared. Enjoy the exotic brightness and interesting layers.

When making the dressing, take the time to sample the flavors—the sourness of the lime and the saltiness of the soy sauce, for example. Remember to use as many of your senses as possible. As the ingredients warm, smell the sweet comforting marmalade and spicy chile.

Really look at the salad ingredients while you are preparing them. Notice texture and color. What does the food feel like? Is it hard or soft? Grainy or sticky? Moist or dry? Enjoy the sound and sensation of chopping different shapes and surfaces. Crush a herb leaf in your fingers. Does that release the aroma? How do the scallions contrast with the sweet, peppery mango?

As you toss the salad in the dressing, notice how the ingredients combine to make a different set of textures and smells.

Take small mouthfuls and at least two minutes to finish each one. Chew as slowly as possible to give yourself time to experience each sensation. Close your eyes and concentrate on the smell, the taste, and the texture.

Notice the peanuts, the way they crunch and crumble in your mouth. How does the saltiness of the soy sauce bring out the sweet flavor burst of a cherry tomato? What is your favorite ingredient? Do you like the chile kick or the freshness of the Lebanese cucumber? Notice if the intensity of the flavors change, and concentrate on the sensation of swallowing.

thai veg salad

Calories per serving 180 • Serves 4
Preparation time 10 minutes, plus cooling • Cooking time 2 minutes

8 oz **cherry tomatoes,**
  quartered
1 **Lebanese cucumber,**
  thinly sliced
1 **green papaya** or **green
  mango**
1 large **red chile,** seeded and
  thinly sliced
1½ cups **bean sprouts**
4 **scallions,** thinly sliced
small handful of **Thai basil
  leaves**
small handful of **mint leaves**
small handful of **fresh cilantro
  leaves**
4 tablespoons **unsalted
  peanuts,** roughly chopped

Chili dressing
2 tablespoons **sweet chili
  sauce**
2 tablespoons **light soy sauce**
2 tablespoons **lime juice**
2 tablespoons **lime
  marmalade**

Make the dressing. Put all the
ingredients in a small saucepan and
warm over low heat, stirring, until
combined. Let cool.

Put the tomatoes, cucumber, papaya or
mango, chile, bean sprouts, scallions,
and herbs in a bowl. Add the dressing and
toss well. Transfer to a platter. Sprinkle
over the peanuts and serve immediately.

Smell

Our sense of smell is more closely related to how things taste than any other sense; 75 percent of what we perceive as taste comes from our sense of smell. When we say a meal tasted good, we might not know that a great part of this is due to our experience of its smell.

When we put food in our mouth, odor molecules from the food travel to olfactory receptor cells at the top of the nasal cavity, which sits just beneath the brain. The olfactory bulb is part of the brain's limbic system, also called the emotional brain. The olfactory bulb has access to the amygdala, which processes emotion, and the hippocampus, which is responsible for associative learning. When we have a cold, we can't taste much. This is due to the buildup of mucus in our nasal passage preventing the odor molecules from reaching the olfactory receptor cells. The brain receives no signal and we experience the food as tasteless. Thus when the sense of smell doesn't work, the sense of taste is not triggered. When children are made to eat food or take medicine they don't like, or that tastes bitter, they hold their nose and gulp it down fast to avoid tasting it.

Why is smell so significant? The sense of smell is thought to be linked to the instinct for survival. When we were cave people, it was important to sniff out danger, such as smoke or fire, rotten food or, on the positive side, a mating partner. Smell is all around us; it enters our body even if we are not aware of it, and we emanate it. Have you ever sat around a campfire? The entire body smells of it. Think of the smell of what we have eaten, such as garlic, or the smell of sweat after sports training. There is even a smell archive in Berlin, managed by Sissel Tolaas, a Norwegian. It opened in 1990 and has 6,763 distinctive smells from all over the world.

Smell can bring back a flood of memories and has a very powerful effect on mood and emotion. (Beware if you are an emotional eater. Chapter 4 "No breath, no life" has more on the influence of emotions on food intake.) Our emotional repertoire can remind us of characteristic smells associated with places and activities in the past. For example, the smell of strong disinfectant can remind you of hospital visits you made as a child. If you encounter that smell later in life, it can trigger feelings of loneliness and abandonment. Have you ever considered that aspect of smell? Are there any smells that nourish you and others that deplete you?

To become open to new and different smells can not only enrich our experience of food and beverages, but also teach us tolerance, and free us from prejudice toward certain smells. For example, durians (fruits from Malaysia) smell rotten. The durian is shaped like a honeydew melon and has sharp thorns. Its flavor is most beguiling but because of its off-putting aroma many people don't even ever try it. In Hong Kong and Thailand it is forbidden to carry this fruit on the subway or bring it into a hotel room.

RECIPES TO EXPLORE SMELL

chile & cilantro fish parcel

Calories per serving 127 • Serves 1
Preparation time 15 minutes, plus marinating and chilling
Cooking time 15 minutes

4½ oz **cod, coley,** or **haddock fillet**
2 teaspoons **lemon juice**
1 tablespoon **fresh cilantro leaves**
1 **garlic clove**
1 **green chile**, seeded and chopped
¼ teaspoon **sugar**
2 teaspoons **plain yogurt**

Place the fish in a nonmetallic dish and sprinkle with the lemon juice. Cover and leave in the refrigerator to marinate for 15–20 minutes.

Put the cilantro, garlic, and chile in a food processor or blender and process until the mixture forms a paste. Add the sugar and yogurt and briefly process to blend.

Lay the fish on a sheet of foil. Coat the fish on both sides with the paste. Gather up the foil loosely and turn over at the top to seal. Return to the refrigerator for at least 1 hour.

Place the parcel on a baking sheet and bake in a preheated oven, 400°F, for about 15 minutes until the fish is just cooked through.

AWARENESS POINTS
- Smell a fresh cilantro leaf and mark its intensity. How does this change after the mixture has been blended in the food processor?
- Does the fish you have chosen remind you of the seaside? Is the smell bringing back any childhood memories?
- When you eat the meal, see if the hot chile has an effect on the nasal passages? Are the smells heightened as a result?

lemon & cardamom madeleines

Calories per serving 80 • Makes about 30
Preparation time 20 minutes, plus setting • Cooking time 30 minutes

9 tablespoons **lightly salted butter**, melted, plus extra for greasing
1 cup **self-rising flour**, plus extra for dusting
2 teaspoons **cardamom pods**
3 **eggs**
⅔ cup **superfine sugar**
finely grated rind of 1 **lemon**
½ teaspoon **baking powder**

Glaze
2 tablespoons **lemon juice**
½ cup + 2 tablespoons **confectioners' sugar**, sifted, plus extra for dusting

Grease a madeleine tray with melted butter and dust with flour. Tap out the excess flour.

Crush the cardamom pods using a mortar and pestle to release the seeds. Remove the shells and crush the seeds a little further.

Put the eggs, superfine sugar, lemon rind, and crushed cardamom seeds in a heatproof bowl and rest the bowl over a saucepan of gently simmering water. Whisk with a handheld electric whisk until the mixture is thick and pale and the whisk leaves a trail when lifted.

Sift the flour and baking powder into the bowl and gently fold in using a large metal spoon. Drizzle the melted butter around the edges of the mixture and fold the ingredients together to combine. Spoon the mixture into the madeleine sections until about two-thirds full. (Keep the remaining mixture for a second batch.)

Bake in a preheated oven, 425°F, for about 10 minutes until risen and golden. Leave in the tray for 5 minutes, then transfer to a wire rack.

Make the glaze by putting the lemon juice in a bowl and beating in the confectioners' sugar. Brush over the madeleines and let set. Serve lightly dusted with confectioners' sugar.

AWARENESS POINTS

- Cardamom seeds are intensely aromatic when crushed. Green pods are sweet flavored and are used in making Garam Masala Chai. Black pods have a smokier aroma.
- Notice the fresh, zingy smell of the lemon before and after you grate the rind.
- The smell of baking is one of the most comforting and appetizing. Use the 30 minutes baking time to savor positive feelings and make sure you savor the eating experience just as much.

Sight

Sight is a trigger for appetite and does not affect the ability to taste, although it influences our perception of taste. For example, some studies show that a darker color makes us think a drink is stronger. When food looks fresh and is well presented, it triggers our taste buds and saliva glands. A well-presented buffet leads us to anticipate a tasty meal. If the buffet looks drab, the salad is limp, and the food is colorless, we are less inclined to have positive expectations.

The main reason for sight's influence is memory of past experiences with color and flavor. We remember what fresh bread looks like compared with moldy bread. We can identify vegetables and fruits that are fresh, those that are past their best, and those that are unripe. We go for the yellow banana, not the green. We choose the brown/green apple for sour taste, the red apple for sweet taste.

Memory influences our food choices. If we have had a good experience with certain food, we think it looks good. If we have no experience with it, our mind will try to associate it with something familiar. We might avoid a specific food because we don't recognize it and it looks strange, weird even, and not very appetizing. We might think we know how it tastes just by looking at it. But we might be mistaken.

If you are hungry, the mind recognizes the overriding need for food and makes you select something, even if it doesn't look that enticing. So try something that looks unfamiliar to you. Maybe some durian? You might feel better because you stepped out of autopilot, happier and empowered. Feeling happier means you can make better choices.

Tip

If the candy bar or potato chip package is left on the coffee table in front of the TV, chances are you won't resist. Put it away and replace it with some healthier options, such as carrot sticks, or apples and grapes with cheese. Remember, out of sight is out of mind. Put healthy food in a prime position; ideally, unhealthy food should be hidden.

tomato & mozzarella salad

Calories per serving 212 • Serves 4
Preparation time 15 minutes

1 lb 2 oz ripe **tomatoes,**
  preferably different types,
  such as heirloom and cherry
  and plum
about 3 tablespoons **olive oil**
2 tablespoons **aged balsamic
  vinegar**
small handful of **basil leaves**
5 oz **mini mozzarella balls**
salt and **black pepper**

Cut half the tomatoes into thick slices and the other half into wedges. Arrange the slices on a large serving plate, slightly overlapping each other.

Put the tomato wedges in a bowl and drizzle with most of the olive oil and balsamic vinegar. Season to taste with salt and pepper. Mix carefully and arrange on top of the tomato slices.

Add the basil leaves and mozzarella balls to the tomato wedges. Drizzle the salad with more olive oil and balsamic vinegar, season to taste with salt and black pepper, and serve.

AWARENESS POINTS
- Make it your mission to choose as many different tomatoes as possible—homegrown or store-bought, you can create a full spectrum of red colors.
- Notice the way the balsamic dressing coats and sinks into the intricate tears in the mozzarella. Imagine how it will add to the flavor.
- Think about presentation. Serve this salad to a friend and notice how the layering of ingredients adds to the impression of the dish.

spring minestrone

Calories per serving 221 • Serves 4
Preparation time 15 minutes • Cooking time 55 minutes

2 tablespoons **olive oil**, plus
extra to serve
1 **onion**, thinly sliced
2 **carrots**, peeled and diced
2 **celery stalks**, diced
2 **garlic cloves**, peeled
1 **potato**, peeled and diced
1 cup **peas** or **fava beans**,
thawed if frozen
1 **zucchini**, diced
4½ oz **green beans**, trimmed
and cut into 1½ inch pieces
4½ oz **plum tomatoes**, skinned
and chopped
5 cups **vegetable stock**
3 oz **small pasta shapes**
10 **basil leaves**, torn
salt and **black pepper**
grated **Parmesan cheese**, to
serve

Heat the oil in a large, heavy-bottomed saucepan over low heat, add the onion, carrots, celery, and garlic, and cook, stirring occasionally, for 10 minutes. Add the potato, peas or fava beans, zucchini, and green beans and cook, stirring frequently, for 2 minutes. Add the tomatoes, season with salt and black pepper, and cook for another 2 minutes.

Pour in the stock and bring to a boil, then reduce the heat and simmer gently for 20 minutes or until all the vegetables are very tender.

Add the pasta and basil to the soup and cook, stirring frequently, until the pasta is al dente. Season with salt and black pepper to taste.

Ladle into bowls, drizzle with olive oil, and sprinkle with the Parmesan. Serve with toasted country bread, if liked.

AWARENESS POINTS
• Watch the texture of this soup change from a broth when it is thickened with stock and the pasta is added. Let this help you to appreciate how filling and nourishing it will be.
• When you tear a basil leaf, examine it in detail—the lines on the leaves and the waxy texture.
• How green is your finished soup? What percentage of green vegetables can you see in your bowl? Do you associate this color with health?

Sound

Food comes with its own sounds. Think of those we make when we are eating—we chomp, crunch, grind, gulp, gnaw, munch, slurp, sputter, choke maybe, burp even. The crunchiness of potato chips, for example, has become an essential part of our enjoyment of them, and our perception of them as fresh. We think the louder they crunch, the fresher the chips.

The sound of calming music can make you feel peaceful and relaxed, and encourage you to stay longer at a restaurant and order another drink, or possibly a dessert. Even if you know that, I guess you may not know that sound can modulate taste, so that food tastes sweeter or more bitter, depending on the music you are listening to. Welcome to the science of "sonic seasoning."

Sound travels to us, but mostly we don't notice. We are busy talking, reading the newspaper or e-mails, or we are on the phone, so we don't notice the sound around us. Sound reaches us, though, whether we are aware of it or not, but we can only hear it if we are tuned in to it. Our auditory system has an extraordinary capacity for conveying information. We might think that sound has little or no impact on our eating habits, but think twice. What about the sound of the sizzling sausage in the pan, the sound of hot water boiling for the first cup of tea, the gurgling sound of the coffee machine, the crunchy potato chips, the sound of nuts cracking, the squelchy sound of a ripe peach?

Our brain recognizes the food by remembering the sounds of food we have eaten in the past. It recognizes loudness, pitch, and type, and once it has confirmed the memory of the sound, it will begin to fire up the part of the brain that desires the item ... Could it be chocolate?

Did you ever wonder why airline food doesn't taste that nice? A study published in 2011 found that loud background noise suppresses saltiness, sweetness, and the overall enjoyment of food. High altitude also blocks the nasal passage and therefore access to aromas. Heston Blumenthal, who devised a menu for BA, mentioned during a TV interview that he always insisted on "over-seasoning airline food" because of the effects of altitude and noise on taste. In future, sound will play a bigger part in our eating experience.

peach & blueberry crunch

Calories per serving 371 • Serves 4 • Preparation time 10 minutes, plus cooling • Cooking time 8–10 minutes

¼ cup **ground hazelnuts**
¼ cup **ground almonds**
2 tablespoons **superfine sugar**
½ cup **bread crumbs**
13½ oz **can peaches** in natural juice
¾ cup **blueberries**
⅔ cup **heavy cream**
seeds from 1 **vanilla bean**
1 tablespoon **confectioners' sugar**, sifted

Gently cook the ground nuts in a large skillet with the sugar and bread crumbs, stirring constantly until golden. Remove from the heat and let cool.

Put the peaches in a food processor or blender and blend with enough of the peach juice to make a thick, smooth puree.

Set aside some of the blueberries to decorate and fold the remaining blueberries gently into the puree. Spoon into 4 glasses or individual serving dishes.

Whip the cream with the vanilla seeds and confectioners' sugar until thick but not stiff and spoon evenly over the peach puree. When the crunchy topping is cool, sprinkle it over the blueberry mixture, top with the remaining blueberries, and serve.

AWARENESS POINTS
- Apply the raisin practice (see page 20) to an almond. When you slowly eat the almond, where can you hear the crunch, in what parts of your head and ears?
- What noise do the ground nuts make in the skillet? Do they hiss or rustle when the pan is shaken?
- How does the creaminess of the blueberry mixture affect the sound of the nuts when you eat them?

sizzling asian lamb burgers

Calories per serving 480 • Serves 4
Preparation time 20 minutes • Cooking time 30 minutes

2 **garlic cloves**, crushed
1 **lemon grass stalk**, finely
 chopped
1 oz **fresh ginger root**, peeled
 and grated
large handful of **fresh cilantro**,
 roughly chopped
1 **hot red chile**, seeded and
 thinly sliced
1 lb 2 oz **lean ground lamb**
2 tablespoons **sunflower oil**
1 small **cucumber**
1 bunch of **scallions**
7 oz **bok choy**
3 tablespoons **light brown
 sugar**
finely grated rind of 2 **limes**,
 plus 4 tablespoons juice
2 tablespoons **fish sauce**
⅓ cup **roasted peanuts**
salt

Blend the garlic, lemon grass, ginger, cilantro, chile, and a little salt in a food processor to make a thick paste. Add the lamb and blend until mixed. Tip out onto the counter and divide the mixture into 4 pieces. Roll each into a ball and flatten into a burger shape.

Heat the oil in a sturdy roasting pan and fry the burgers on both sides to sear. Transfer to a preheated oven, 400°F, and cook, uncovered, for 25 minutes until the burgers are cooked through.

Meanwhile, peel the cucumber and cut in half lengthwise. Scoop out the seeds with a teaspoon and discard. Cut the cucumber into thin, diagonal slices. Slice the scallions diagonally. Roughly shred the bok choy; keep the white parts separate from the green.

Using a large metal spoon, drain off all but about 2 tablespoons fat from the roasting pan. Arrange all the vegetables except the green parts of the bok choy around the meat and toss them gently in the pan juices. Return to the oven, uncovered, for 5 minutes.

Mix together the sugar, lime rind and juice, and fish sauce. Scatter the bok choy greens and peanuts into the roasting pan and drizzle with half the dressing.

Toss the salad ingredients together gently. Transfer the lamb and salad to serving plates and drizzle with the remaining dressing.

AWARENESS POINTS
- Notice how the sound of the oil can trigger an inbuilt warning of danger, encouraging you to be extra careful when cooking.
- What noise do the burgers make when they hit the pan?
- As you tear the bok choy, notice which parts of the vegetable are the crispest.

Touch

Touch is integral to our experience with food. It informs us about texture, moisture, chewiness, greasiness, whether the food is likely to be painful (hot chile), or astringent. By touching we know if a peach is ripe or not, we sense the smoothness of the apple, the roughness of the pear, the waxed surface of the lemon/orange, we feel if the food is heavy or light, hot or cold, wet or dry. All this information is carried to the brain where it is assessed, stimulating desire or dislike, so that we know to wait for the drink to cool down, or the peach to ripen before eating it.

Touch influences our perception of taste, too. Bread that is hard, even if the taste and smell are okay, is not pleasant. We won't eat cold oatmeal; some people don't like lukewarm milk or the spiky feeling of the edible cactus.

baked figs with goat cheese

Calories per serving 201 • Serves 4
Preparation time 10 minutes • Cooking time 10–12 minutes

8 firm but ripe **fresh figs**
3 oz **soft goat cheese**
8 **mint leaves**
2 tablespoons **extra virgin olive oil**
salt and **pepper**

Arugula salad
5 oz **baby arugula leaves**
1 tablespoon **extra virgin olive oil**
1 teaspoon **lemon juice**

Cut a cross in the top of each fig without cutting through the base. Put 1 teaspoonful of the goat cheese and a mint leaf in each fig. Transfer to a roasting pan, then season with salt and pepper and drizzle with the oil.

Bake in a preheated oven, 375°F, for 10–12 minutes until the figs are soft and the cheese has melted.

Make the arugula salad. Put the baby arugula leaves in a bowl. Whisk together the oil, lemon juice, salt, and pepper in a small bowl and drizzle over the leaves. Serve with the figs.

AWARENESS POINTS
- Are the figs hard or soft? When you cut them open, how does the inside texture feel compared to the outside?
- Notice the ease with which you can spoon goat cheese compared to the force needed to cut through a fruit skin.
- How do the warm figs complement the cold arugula salad?

layered nutty bars

Calories per serving 406 • Cuts into 10
Preparation time 20 minutes, plus chilling • Cooking time 5 minutes

3½ tablespoons **butter**
1¾ cups **fat-free sweetened condensed milk**
7 oz **semisweet chocolate**, broken into pieces
4½ oz **sweet tea cookies**
⅓ cup **hazelnuts**
⅔ cup **pistachios**, shelled

Use a little of the butter to grease the bottom and sides of an 8 inch round springform pan. Put the remaining butter in a saucepan with the condensed milk and chocolate. Heat gently for 3–4 minutes, stirring until melted, then remove from the heat.

Place the cookies in a plastic bag and crush roughly into chunky pieces using a rolling pin. Toast the hazelnuts under a preheated hot broiler until lightly browned, then roughly chop with the pistachios.

Stir the cookies into the chocolate mixture, then spoon half the mixture into the prepared pan and spread level. Set aside 2 tablespoons of the nuts for the top, then sprinkle the rest over the cookie layer. Cover with the remaining chocolate mixture, level the surface with the back of the spoon, and sprinkle with the reserved nuts.

Chill the nut mixture for 3–4 hours until firm, then loosen the edges and remove the sides of the pan. Cut into 10 thin slices, or into tiny bite-size pieces to make petits fours.

AWARENESS POINTS
• This baking recipe is great for getting your hands messy and really connecting with the food.
• Use clean hands to grease the pan, noticing the coolness of the metal.
• As you add each layer of nuts and cookies to the pan, carefully push into place with your fingers, exploring and comparing the rough textures.

Taste

Flavor is important to us and what we call taste is the interconnected experience of several senses, especially smell and touch, into one single experience. When we put food into our mouth, the taste receptors on the tongue and the roof of the mouth (the taste buds) send an impulse to the brain through the cranial nerve. The brain then compares the information with stored memory of previous tastes and recognizes what you are eating. After that, it will decide if you like the taste of the food or drink, and if it is a good idea to continue consuming it.

We used to refer to four tastes—sweet, bitter, sour, and salty—but recently another one, umami, has been recognized. This is found in fermented and aged foods, such as cheese and tamari (a variety of soy sauce from Japan), and is savory.

It was once thought that these tastes were centered on different areas of the tongue but this is now no longer considered to be true. Each taste bud, no matter where it sits on the tongue, has the potential to pick up any of the five known tastes.

flourless chocolate cake—bitter

Calories per serving 488 • Cuts into 12
Preparation time 25 minutes • Cooking time 1 hour

scant 1 cup **blanched almonds,**
  roughly chopped
scant 1 cup **Brazil nuts,**
  roughly chopped
7½ oz **semisweet chocolate,**
  chopped into ¼ inch pieces
½ lb (2 sticks) **slightly salted**
  butter, softened
4 **eggs,** separated
generous 1 cup **superfine**
  sugar
sifted **unsweetened cocoa,**
  for dusting

Put the nuts and chocolate in a food processor and process until ground. Beat together the butter, yolks, and generous ¾ cup of the sugar in a bowl until pale and creamy. Stir in the chocolate mixture.

Whisk the egg whites in a large clean bowl with a handheld electric whisk until peaking. Gradually whisk in the remaining sugar, a spoonful at a time. Stir a quarter of the mixture into the creamed mixture using a large metal spoon. Add the remaining whites and stir gently to mix.

Spoon the mixture into a greased and lined 9 inch loose-bottomed or springform cake pan and level the surface. Bake in a preheated oven, 325°F, for about 1 hour or until just firm to the touch afnd a skewer inserted into the center comes out clean.

Let cool in the pan (the cake's center will sink slightly), then remove the ring and bottom and dust with sifted cocoa.

AWARENESS POINT
• Before you mix the cake ingredients, place a very small piece of chopped semisweet chocolate on the tip of your tongue. Close your eyes, and let the chocolate melt in your mouth. Mark all the sensations and try to pinpoint where in the mouth you taste the bitterness.

warm chicken salad with anchovies—salty

Calories per serving 303 • Serves 4
Preparation time 20 minutes • Cooking time 15–17 minutes

5 oz **green beans**, trimmed
and thickly sliced
1 small crisp **lettuce**, leaves
separated and torn into
pieces
6 **scallions**, thinly sliced
6 oz **cherry tomatoes**, halved
9 oz jar **mixed pepper
antipasto in oil**
2 **boneless, skinless chicken
breasts**, diced
1 cup **fresh bread crumbs**
4 canned **anchovy fillets**,
drained and chopped

Dressing
3 tablespoons **olive oil**
2 teaspoons **sun-dried tomato
paste**
4 teaspoons **red wine vinegar**
salt and **black pepper**

Blanch the green beans in a saucepan
of boiling water for 3–4 minutes until just
tender. Drain, rinse with cold water, and
drain again.

Put the beans, lettuce, scallions, and
tomatoes into a large salad bowl. Lift the
peppers out of the jar, reserving the oil,
dice if needed, and add to the salad.

Pour 2 tablespoons of the oil from the
pepper jar into a skillet, add the chicken,
and fry for 8–10 minutes, stirring until
golden and cooked through. Spoon over
the salad. Heat another 1 tablespoon of
the oil in the pan, add the bread crumbs
and anchovies and stir-fry until golden.

Mix the dressing ingredients together,
toss over the salad, then sprinkle with
the bread crumbs and anchovies and
serve immediately.

AWARENESS POINT
• Chopping and preparing fish is not everyone's favorite kitchen pastime, but
when you open the can of anchovies, take a small bite of one and focus on the
kick of the salty taste rather than the smell. A salad is a great way to explore
your senses as you never quite know what taste combination you're going to
get. Count and mark how salty every bite is on a very rough scale of, say, one
to three. What do you enjoy? What is too much? How does the salt bring out
the other flavors, and was the salt necessary?

fig & honey pots—sweet

Calories per serving 260 • Serves 4
Preparation time 10 minutes, plus chilling

6 ripe **fresh figs**, thinly sliced,
  plus 2 extra, cut into wedges,
  to decorate (optional)
2 cups **whole Greek yogurt**
4 tablespoons **clear honey**
2 tablespoons **pistachios**,
  chopped

Arrange the fig slices snugly in the bottom of 4 glasses or glass bowls. Spoon the yogurt over the figs and chill in the refrigerator for 10–15 minutes.

Just before serving, drizzle 1 tablespoon honey over each dessert and sprinkle the pistachios on top. Decorate with the fig wedges, if liked.

AWARENESS POINT
• Most diets encourage you to go for natural sugars rather than artificial sweeteners, and honey is one of the best sources. Not only that, but it comes in a wide variety of flavors, so you can have a richer, deeper experience when it comes to those sweet cravings. Why not treat yourself to a mini honey tasting—smear a small amount of each flavor onto a plain cracker and try to describe the different taste sensations.

crab & grapefruit salad—sour

Calories per serving 384 • Serves 4
Preparation time 10 minutes

13 oz **white crabmeat**
1 **pink grapefruit**, peeled and sliced
2 oz **arugula leaves**
3 **scallions**, sliced
7 oz **snow peas**, halved
salt and **black pepper**

Watercress dressing
3¼ oz **watercress**, tough stalks removed
1 tablespoon **Dijon mustard**
2 tablespoon **olive oil**

To serve
4 **chapattis**
lime wedges

Combine the crabmeat, grapefruit, arugula, scallions, and snow peas in a serving dish. Season to taste.

Make the dressing by blending together the watercress, mustard, and oil. Season with salt.

Toast the chapattis. Stir the dressing into the salad and serve with the toasted chapattis and lime wedges on the side.

AWARENESS POINT
• Grapefruit is one of the sharpest ingredients known. Love it or hate it, a grapefruit is a ritual to cut open and eat. The sheer bright pink color alerts the brain to a strong taste. Eat a few segments while you make this salad. Where do you taste the sourness? What physical sensations occur?

2 The intelligent body

"Those who know when they have enough will not be disgraced;
Those who know how to stop will not be harmed."
LAO TZU

Food heaven

In 2007 Mireille Guiliano unveiled the secret of eating for pleasure in her book, catchily titled *French Women Don't Get Fat*. Have you ever visited France and been tempted by delicious breads and patisserie, cheese and wine? Do you go straight to your favorite little café and order *café au lait et un croissant*? Perhaps you breathe in the scrumptious smell of fresh coffee and buttery baked heaven and dunk the latter into the former and receive the gift from the gods. Simply fabulous! Or what about a memory of a long, celebratory meal? Imagine a banquet when course after course appears, conversation is unhurried and tempered so it's enjoyable but does not distract from the wonderful eating experience. Did you appreciate the time to digest while plates were cleared and the next dish took its time to arrive?

French food makes you mindful, if you haven't yet grasped the concept. So what is it that they are doing differently?

As Mireille Guiliano suggests in her book, the French don't get fat because they know how to eat and when to stop eating. How do they know? Research suggests that they pay more attention to internal cues, such as whether they feel full, and less attention to external cues, such as the potato chip bag is empty. They rarely have to loosen their belt by two holes. One other major factor is time—lunchbreaks last anything between one and two hours.

Lost in autopilot

It seems that we have lost the ability to feel the signals the body is sending us to indicate that it is full. The body does not require calorie tables, because it knows perfectly well when to stop. Does the following sound familiar?

"I don't know any more when I'm hungry or full up. I have been on too many diets and I don't know how to listen to my body's messages. I remember that when I was a child, I ate when I was hungry and stopped when I'd had enough and rushed out to play again with my friends. But dieting made me ignore my belly's hunger signals and I started eating according to the calorie tables I was given."

Paying attention to bodily sensations is a central part of mindful eating. As we increase our awareness, we learn to read the signs and to stop when we are full. Being in your body means you are in the present moment. It is in the now that you can feel your hunger. Unfortunately, people often eat for the future. Some people say they were eating even when they were not hungry, just to make sure they would not be hungry later in the day. By getting in touch with the body, you will relearn how it feels when you are hungry and when you are full.

By paying attention to the body, we change our relationship with it. We stop trying to control it and befriend it instead. We start to care for it. By paying attention to it, we make it special. In *The Little Prince* by Antoine de Saint-Exupéry, the rose is special because the little prince cared for it.

The loss of innocence

Our relationship with our bodies has become complicated. We are judgmental, especially regarding image and shape—the body is ugly, disgusting, loathsome, yuk, frumpy, a blob, sordid, weak—and it is not only our own condemnatory thoughts that have estranged us from our bodies. We listen to other people talking and as we feel rejected, so we reject ourselves. By talking to ourselves like this, we miss hearing or sensing our body's subtle voice. Relearning to take notice of a light pressure in the stomach or some slight difficulty breathing as we get fuller is one of the most important goals in rebalancing our weight. Occasionally, our body's voice gets louder, or even screams. We may be feeling sick, overfull, uncomfortable. We have problems with digestion, develop heartburn. How loud does it need to get? Unfortunately, most of us, most of the time, are not truly present in our bodies.

It wasn't always like this. There was a time when we didn't even think about our body, let alone judge it. We just lived in it. In our childhood we were bundles of energy, open, vulnerable, and vibrating. The body had not yet been fragmented into parts that we judged separately. It didn't matter what we looked like. We didn't worry about our basic needs or how to fulfill them. The body and its innate intelligence took care of it. We slept when we were tired, and we cried when we needed food or cuddles. Our body was tirelessly and reliably working for us and supporting us as it was turning food into blood, bones, and tissue. That is what we call the intelligence of the original body.

You may wonder what causes the loss of this simple and straightforward relationship with our body that was once a natural part of life. The answer is simple and yet hard to believe. The loss occurs through the process of growing up and being taught about "civilized" behavior, including how we should walk, sit, conduct ourselves, and dress according to our gender, age, class, and culture. As we start to look after ourselves, our relationship with our body changes. We want to feel safe, and overprotect the body so that it becomes contracted, tighter, and less open and vulnerable. We lose contact with its original nature and begin to observe it as if it is an object. Instead of acknowledging that we are living in this body and that it is essential and deeply connected to what we call "I," we start to distance ourselves from it. We begin to bend it, form it (for example, Chinese foot binding or wearing corsets), encourage it to grow thinner or fatter (depending on the dominant culture), and eventually split it into parts we like and those we dislike. Through this process we stop experiencing our unique, pulsating body and, instead, feel a deep separation from it.

People who work with traumatized patients speak about the body being held in a "frozen frame." The first to investigate this phenomenon was psychologist Wilhelm Reich. He explored the idea that emotional trauma created holding patterns in our body's soft tissue. Furthermore, he discovered that by working with the body, the emotional trauma could be released. Others followed in his footsteps—Ida Rolf, Moshe Feldenkrais, Alexander Lowen, and the founder of Hakomi body-centered therapy, the late Ron Kurtz. What they all have in common is the aim of bringing the body and its sensations back into the field of our awareness so that once again we can feel its natural ability to pulse and flow with life.

Letting go—simply be

"Do nothing with the body but relax"
TILOPA

Pleasant sensations often lead to a wish that they may stay forever. Unpleasant sensations create the desire for them to leave as soon as possible. These thoughts generate tension in our body. Mental patterns of reaction, of clinging or aversion, are physical actions, and no matter how subtle they are, they create muscular tensions. Here is a big lesson to be learned about the arising of suffering—wanting things to be other than the way they are is the root cause of most emotional and even a lot of physical suffering.

Being in your body, learning how to relax, allows the full range of sensations to rise to the surface. If the mind is lost in thought, this thought will be accompanied directly by a muscular contraction somewhere in the body. This tension is calling us back home.

Practices

Here are two variations on the body scan. See which one appeals to you most, or simply experiment with them. Each one takes about 30 minutes but that can be stretched out for longer or, when you have practiced them often enough, shortened. They can be experienced at any time of the day and are a useful tool for making contact with your body. When you listen to your body at times when you feel empty, ask yourself if you are really hungry or if there is an alternative nourishment you may require—going for a walk, listening to music, having a hot bath, connecting with a friend.

Close your eyes, smile, and relax. Remember you are not looking for any particular sensations. You are not trying to make anything particular happen, or change what you are aware of. Focus on whatever comes into your awareness.

There might be sensations of tingling, numbness, warmth, cold, neutrality, pleasantness, or unpleasantness. Areas can feel moist or dry, pulsating, flowing, or itchy. Whatever it is, it is important for you to be aware of it. Be as open and receptive as possible; no need to add anything or take something away.

Try to savor the sensations as if you have attended a wine-tasting session and are sipping some wine that is really special, or you have been served with a meal that is out of this world. You would be totally focused and forget all your worries and plans; you would be fully present. Just be with the sensations that occur. There are no right or wrong sensations. Let go of thinking and just sense them. Kindness is important, too, just sensing what is without any extra effort. What we are talking about here is effortless awareness. The sensation is okay as it is. It is part of the experience. Have the courage and strength to be with what is.

The musical body scan

This practice was taught by the late Gurdjieff. Today, he is mostly forgotten but he was quite extreme in his methods of awakening people. He didn't use the terms mindfulness or mindlessness, but when he spoke of us as the "walking dead," "zombie-like" creatures, he meant the same.

Most of our lives are spent on autopilot. Eating on autopilot will definitely make us put on weight and one technique he suggested to avoid this was the "musical body exercise." You are invited to practice it daily at a time that suits you, and to make it a natural part of your life. This will enable you to establish a firm relationship with your body and so to monitor what is happening with it.

- Choose some smooth, soothing, flowing instrumental music that lasts for about half an hour.
- Make sure you will not be disturbed.
- Lie or sit comfortably and keep warm.
- Listen to the music and feel it in your body, starting with your feet and moving on at roughly one-minute intervals:
  —Right foot, right leg, knee, and upper half of your right leg.
  —Now move to your right hand, right forearm. Savor the experience that you are having in the upper right arm.

—Now move to the upper half of the left arm. Down the elbow to the lower half of the arm, then the left hand. If you drifted off for a moment, just come back, feeling the left hand and the fingers.

—Now move down the upper half of the left leg, then the lower half of the left leg, down into the left foot. Don't worry if sensations of other body parts enter the mind. Notice and come back to feel where you have got to in the progression.

—Now feel both feet and both legs at the same time. Widen the focus even more and feel your legs, feet, arms, and hands at the same time.

—Feel that the legs are linked to the pelvis, and the arms are linked to the ribcage. Feel the legs and arms and your trunk, front and back.

—Feel the line of the spine from tailbone to crown. Feel that the pelvis and legs, the chest, and arms are attached to it … now feel your entire body vibrating with the sound of music.

- Sense and feel the music in your entire body until it ends.
- When everything is still, slowly open your eyes and get up, and maintain a sense of being in your body throughout the day.

The bathrobe body scan

This is a fantastic practice when you are exhausted to such an extent that you are feeling tired all the time. Instead of eating more as a way of coping, what you really need is a good dose of sweet relaxation.

- Carve out some time, up to two hours on your day off. Keep your leggings or your pyjamas on, roll out a soft blanket or your yoga mat, dot lots of comfortable pillows on the floor, and put a "please do not disturb" sign on your door.
- Find a comfortable position lying on your back on the blanket or mat on the floor. You can tuck pillows under your knees and hips, a rolled-up towel under your lower back, and flat pillows under your shoulders and head. All the body areas that are not touching the floor are now supported and you can let go more fully to the pull of gravity. Notice how you are sinking into the ground, the softening of your hold around the belly and the chest. With each out breath feel you sink deeper. Don't worry that you are going to fall asleep. This might be exactly what you need.
- Try to stay comfortable for at least 30 minutes and up to two hours, allowing yourself just to be. During this time you might have moments of drowsiness, with no thoughts at all, interspersed with moments of dreamlike images or thoughts. Try not to engage or judge these events; just stay with the softening, relaxing, and opening of your body. Notice how it feels to be totally relaxed. You are developing the base for a calmer and more receptive you.
- When you feel your energy has returned, slowly sit up.

Guided Practice: Oatmeal with Prune Compote

Start the day as you mean to go on and be as kind to your body as possible. Oats are a good source of slow-release carbohydrates, and oatmeal is something we associate with comfort, warmth, and sharing. You can vary the first recipe here by adding seeds, different fruits, honeys, and syrups—it is a great dish to leave you feeling full and satisfied.

Everyone has their own personal preference when it comes to oatmeal consistency so enjoy the sensation of stirring the milk and watching the oats thicken. Choose your favorite bowl and spoon—perhaps someone gave them to you as a gift, they have strong memories attached or you like the shape and color.

When you sit down to eat, take a moment to assess how your body feels. Register any feelings of tension. Pay attention in turn to your mouth, throat, chest, and stomach. Are you too hot or cold? Do you need to open the window or put on a sweater before you start eating? Is your stomach rumbling? Is the smell of delicious oatmeal making your mouth water? Have you had a glass of water—perhaps you are dehydrated?

Sit up straight, pick up the spoon carefully, and bring one small spoonful to your mouth. Test how hot it is. As you eat the first mouthful, concentrate on the sensation of the oatmeal in your mouth. Is it creamy? Is it coarse? Is the consistency just how you like it? Notice how it warms your throat, down through your chest, and into your stomach.

Recent studies say it takes 20 minutes before we register the feeling of fullness, so take as long to finish as possible. Savor every spoonful. See how the feeling of hunger changes and lessens. Perhaps you don't need to eat the whole bowl of oatmeal? It is all right not to finish your meal; next time you'll know to make a smaller portion. You could try pausing and putting down your spoon between mouthfuls.

Finally, compare how you feel now with when you started your breakfast. Do you feel full and satisfied? Is your body less tense? Enjoy the feeling of being full, but not too full—just right.

oatmeal with prune compote

Calories per serving 259 • Serves 8
Preparation time 5 minutes • Cooking time about 20 minutes

4 cups **skim** or **lowfat milk**
1 teaspoon **vanilla extract**
pinch of **ground cinnamon**
pinch of **salt**
2⅓ cups **porridge oats**
3 tablespoons **slivered almonds**, toasted

Compote
8 oz **ready-to-eat dried Agen prunes**
½ cup **apple juice**
1 small **cinnamon stick**
1 **clove**
1 tablespoon **clear honey**
1 unpeeled **orange** quarter

Place all the compote ingredients in a small saucepan over medium heat. Simmer gently for 10–12 minutes or until softened and slightly sticky. Let cool. (The compote can be prepared in advance and chilled.)

Put the milk, 2 cups water, vanilla extract, cinnamon, and salt in a large saucepan over medium heat and bring slowly to a boil. Stir in the oats, then reduce the heat and simmer gently, stirring occasionally, for 8–10 minutes until creamy and tender.

Spoon the oatmeal into warmed bowls, scatter with the almonds, and serve with the prune compote.

For sweet quinoa oatmeal with banana & dates, put scant 1½ cups quinoa in a saucepan with the milk, 1 tablespoon agave nectar or honey, and 2–3 cardamom pods. Simmer gently for 12–15 minutes or until the quinoa is cooked and the desired consistency is reached. Serve in bowls topped with a dollop of fat-free plain yogurt, 3½ oz chopped dates, and freshly sliced banana.

turkey râgout

Calories per serving 190 • Serves 4
Preparation time 10 minutes • Cooking time 1 hour 50 minutes

1 **turkey drumstick**, about
1¼ lb
2 **garlic cloves**
15 **pearl onions** or **shallots**
3 **carrots**, diagonally sliced
1¼ cups **red wine**
a few **thyme sprigs**
2 **bay leaves**
2 tablespoons chopped **flat-leaf parsley**
1 teaspoon **port wine jelly**
1 teaspoon **wholegrain mustard**
salt and **black pepper**

Carefully remove the skin from the turkey drumstick and make a few cuts in the flesh. Finely slice 1 of the garlic cloves and push the slivers into the slashes. Crush the remaining garlic clove.

Transfer the drumstick to a large, ovenproof casserole, Dutch oven, or roasting pan with the onions or shallots, carrots, crushed garlic, red wine, thyme, and bay leaves.

Season well with salt and black pepper, cover, and place in a preheated oven, 350°F, for about 1¾ hours or until the turkey is cooked through.

Remove the turkey and vegetables from the pan and keep hot. Bring the sauce to a boil on the stove, discarding the bay leaves. Add the parsley, port wine jelly, and mustard. Boil for 5 minutes until slightly thickened. Season with salt and pepper. Carve the turkey and serve with the juices in 4 serving bowls.

AWARENESS POINTS
• Monitor your body sensations before you begin to eat. Pause after five mouthfuls. Has anything changed?
• Can you single out the taste of the mustard? What sensations can you feel in your mouth and stomach?
• Remember what you have learned in the chapter. Protein and carbohydrates will keep you fuller for longer. See if you can distinguish this feeling of fullness compared with the hit of a sugary snack or greasy takeout.

seeded oatcakes

Calories per serving 65 • Makes 20
Preparation time 15 minutes • Cooking time 25 minutes

1½ cups **medium oatmeal**
generous ½ cup **all-purpose flour**, plus extra for dusting
4 tablespoons **mixed seeds**, such as **poppy seeds**, **flaxseeds**, and **sesame seeds**
½ teaspoon **celery salt** or **sea salt**
½ teaspoon freshly ground **black pepper**
3½ tablespoons **unsalted butter**, chilled and diced, plus extra for greasing
5 tablespoons **cold water**

Put the oatmeal, flour, seeds, salt, and black pepper in a bowl or food processor. Add the butter and rub in with the fingertips or process until the mixture resembles bread crumbs. Add the measurement water and mix or blend to a firm dough, adding a little more water if the dough feels dry.

Roll out the dough on a lightly floured counter to ⅛ inch thick. Cut out 20 circles using a 2½ inch plain or fluted cookie cutter, rerolling the trimmings to make more. Place slightly apart on a large greased baking sheet.

Bake in a preheated oven, 350°F, for about 25 minutes until firm. Transfer to a wire rack to cool. Serve with cheese, if liked.

AWARENESS POINTS
• Notice the feel of the bread crumb mixture in your fingers when you make the dough.
• Choose a number of oatcakes per portion. Pause between each oatcake and avoid the temptation to go for more just because they are there.
• Take small bites and compare the coarse texture of the oatcake with the crumbling texture of the cheese.

white bean soup provençal

Calories per serving 200 (not including crusty bread) • Serves 6
Preparation time 15 minutes, plus overnight soaking
Cooking time 1¼–1¾ hours

3 tablespoons **olive oil**

2 **garlic cloves**, crushed

1 small **red bell pepper**, cored, seeded, and chopped

1 **onion**, finely chopped

8 oz **tomatoes**, finely chopped

1 teaspoon finely chopped **thyme**

2¼ cups **dried haricot** or **cannellini beans**, soaked overnight in cold water, rinsed, and drained

2½ cups **water**

2½ cups **vegetable stock**

2 tablespoons finely chopped **flat-leaf parsley**

salt and **black pepper**

Heat the oil in a large heavy-bottomed saucepan, add the garlic, red bell pepper, and onion and cook over medium heat for 5 minutes or until softened.

Add the tomatoes and thyme and cook for 1 minute. Add the beans and pour in the measurement water and stock. Bring to a boil, then reduce the heat, cover, and simmer for 1–1½ hours until the beans are tender (you may need to allow for a longer cooking time, depending on how old the beans are).

Sprinkle in the parsley and season with salt and black pepper. Ladle into warm soup bowls and serve immediately with fresh, crusty bread, if liked.

AWARENESS POINTS

• How does the smell of the soup affect your appetite?

• Think etiquette—try sipping, not slurping.

• Notice the warmth of the soup as it travels from your mouth to your throat and stomach.

butternut squash & ricotta frittata

Calories per serving 248 • Serves 6
Preparation time 10 minutes • Cooking time 25–30 minutes

1 tablespoon **extra virgin canola oil**
1 **red onion**, thinly sliced
14½ oz peeled **butternut squash**, diced
8 **eggs**
1 tablespoon chopped **thyme**
2 tablespoons chopped **sage**
½ cup **ricotta cheese**
salt and **black pepper**

Heat the oil in a large, deep skillet with an ovenproof handle over medium-low heat, add the onion and butternut squash, then cover loosely and cook gently, stirring frequently, for 18–20 minutes or until softened and golden.

Lightly beat the eggs, thyme, sage, and ricotta in a pitcher, then season well with salt and pepper and pour over the squash.

Cook for another 2–3 minutes until the egg is almost set, stirring occasionally with a heat-resistant rubber spatula to prevent the base from burning.

Slide the pan under a preheated broiler, keeping the handle away from the heat, and broil for 3–4 minutes or until the egg is set and the frittata is golden. Slice into 6 wedges and serve hot.

AWARENESS POINTS
- Try to work this in to your lunch menu as an alternative to stodgy sandwiches.
- Appreciate the complexity of the ingredients and the science behind them. When you beat the ingredients, how do they combine?
- Look at the layers of the frittata and imagine your stomach slowly filling up, layer upon layer.

turkish lamb & spinach curry

Calories per serving 497 • Serves 4
Preparation time 20 minutes • Cooking time 2 hours

4 tablespoons **sunflower oil**
1¼ lb **boneless shoulder of lamb**, cut into bite-size pieces
1 **onion**, finely chopped
3 **garlic cloves**, crushed
1 teaspoon **ground ginger**
2 teaspoons **ground turmeric**
large pinch of **grated nutmeg**
4 tablespoons **golden raisins**
1 teaspoon **ground cinnamon**
1 teaspoon **paprika**
13 oz can **chopped tomatoes**
1¼ cups **lamb stock**
13 oz **baby leaf spinach**
salt and **black pepper**

Heat half the oil in a large, heavy-bottomed saucepan and brown the lamb, in batches, for 3–4 minutes. Remove with a slotted spoon and set aside.

Put the remaining oil in the pan and add the onion, garlic, ginger, turmeric, nutmeg, golden raisins, cinnamon, and paprika. Stir-fry for 1–2 minutes, then add the lamb. Stir-fry for another 2–3 minutes, then add the tomatoes and stock. Season well and bring to a boil.

Reduce the heat, cover tightly, and simmer very gently (using a heat diffuser if possible) for 1½ hours.

Add the spinach in batches until it is all wilted, cover, and cook for another 10–12 minutes, stirring occasionally. Remove from the heat and serve drizzled with whisked yogurt, if liked.

AWARENESS POINTS
• Get to know your spices. Could you identify them in a line-up?
• How does the lamb change color as it cooks? When is the meat just the right juicy texture?
• Try to distinguish the ginger and the nutmeg as you chew and eventually swallow each small mouthful.

salmon & puy lentils with parsley

Calories per serving 486 • Serves 4
Preparation time 15 minutes • Cooking time 35 minutes

1 cup **Puy lentils**
1 **bay leaf**
7 oz **fine green beans**, chopped
½ cup **flat-leaf parsley**,
  chopped
2 tablespoons **Dijon mustard**
2 tablespoons **capers**, rinsed
  and chopped
2 tablespoons **olive oil**
2 **lemons**, finely sliced
about 1 lb 2 oz **salmon fillets**
1 **fennel bulb**, finely sliced
salt and **black pepper**
dill weed sprigs, to garnish

Put the lentils into a saucepan with the bay leaf and enough cold water to cover (do not add salt). Bring to a boil, reduce to a simmer, and cook for 30 minutes or until tender. Season to taste, add the beans, and simmer for 1 minute. Drain the lentils and stir in the parsley, mustard, capers, and oil. Discard the bay leaf.

Meanwhile, arrange the lemon slices on a foil-lined broiler pan and put the salmon and fennel slices on top. Season the salmon and fennel and cook under a preheated hot broiler for about 10 minutes or until the salmon is cooked through.

Serve the fennel slices and lentils with the salmon on top, garnished with dill weed sprigs.

AWARENESS POINTS
- What color is your salmon? Can you tell how fresh it is? Do you know its original source?
- This is a fantastic fresh and healthy dish—imagine each mouthful restoring your body with goodness.
- Observe your portion size. Note how choosing the right foods can keep you fuller for longer.

roasted peppers with quinoa

Calories per serving 489 • Serves 4
Preparation time 15 minutes • Cooking time 45 minutes

2 **romano** or **long red bell peppers**, halved, cored, and seeded
20 **red** and **yellow cherry tomatoes**, halved
2 large **yellow bell peppers**, halved, cored, and seeded
1 teaspoon **cumin seeds**
2 tablespoons **olive oil**
generous 1 cup **quinoa**
1 **onion**, finely chopped
½ teaspoon **ground ginger**
1 teaspoon **paprika**
pinch of **grated nutmeg**
generous ¼ cup **ready-to-eat dried apricots**, chopped
2 oz **pitted dates**, chopped
⅓ cup shelled **pistachios**
¼ cup **slivered almonds**, toasted, plus extra to garnish
salt and **black pepper**

Fill the red peppers with the yellow cherry tomatoes and the yellow peppers with the red tomatoes. Scatter over the cumin seeds, drizzle with 1 tablespoon of the oil, and season well with salt and pepper. Place in a preheated oven, 350°F, for about 45 minutes or until tender and slightly blackened around the edges.

Meanwhile, rinse the quinoa several times in cold water. Pour into a pan with twice its volume of boiling water, cover, and simmer for about 12 minutes. It is cooked when the seed is coming away from the germ. Remove from the heat, cover, and let stand until all the water has been absorbed.

Heat the remaining oil in a small skillet over medium heat, add the onion, and cook for 10 minutes or until softened. Add the spices, dried fruits, and nuts, and cook for another 3–4 minutes, or until the fruits have softened, stirring frequently. Gently fold into the cooked quinoa and garnish with the reserved almonds.

AWARENESS POINTS
• Take the time to enjoy the bright colors of the peppers and tomatoes. Do they remind you of anything?
• With over a dozen ingredients in this dish, can you identify each one in the finished dish on your plate?
• How does the texture of the quinoa add to your body's sensations of fullness?

3 Moving with a mindful mind

This chapter is not only for the folks who have "shelved" the whole idea of movement, but also for those who go regularly to the gym and are highly active. Please read on and find out the benefits of mindful movement.

Health data show that a sedentary lifestyle poses a greater risk of heart disease to women over 30 than smoking, obesity, or high blood pressure. Researchers have said that the danger of an inactive lifestyle is being underestimated and deserves to be a much higher public health priority than it has been so far.

Rates of obesity are set to increase in almost every country in Europe throughout the next decade and beyond, with the UK and Ireland among the continent's worst performers. Health authorities anticipate that three in every four men and nearly as many women in the UK will be overweight or obese by 2030. Professor Roberto de Vogli of the University of California said the dominance of supermarkets, high levels of fast-food consumption, and reluctance on the part of government to introduce laws regulating the way food companies make and market their food were all contributing to the US's high obesity rates.

Doesn't sound too encouraging, does it? On the other hand, much of this trouble can be reduced, if not altogether avoided, by bringing some mindful movement back into our lives. Mindful movement can be a way of getting you off the couch, so that you can start enjoying simple activities such as walking again. But the "mindfulness" factor can also be an important addition to an existing workout routine.

Mindful movement

The mindful form of exercise brings you back in touch with your body through movement. The founding father of mindfulness within the secular world, Jon Kabat-Zinn, introduced yoga into his program because he had found it to be very helpful and enjoyable in his own life. As he said in 1990, "The focus is on maintaining moment-to-moment awareness of the sensations accompanying our movements, letting go of any thoughts or feelings about the sensations themselves." By learning to stay with our body sensations as opposed to our thoughts we learn:

- To feel the body from the inside out. This means we learn to know when we are hungry and when we aren't.
- To read the early signs that the body communicates to let us know if we are truly hungry, sated, full, or stuffed.
- To free ourselves from the grip of the thinking mind, the "hungry ghost."
- To move into "being" mode as a way of taking care of our body.

Mindfulness flourishes under what are called the eight attitudinal foundations of mindfulness. Knowing them will help you to differentiate between a normal practice and a mindful movement practice.

The eight attitudinal foundations are:

- Nonjudging
- Patience
- Beginner's mind (childlike curiosity)
- Trust
- Nonstriving
- Acceptance
- Letting go

If your exercise teacher (and remember you are your own teacher when you practice at home) enables you to integrate these elements into your movement practice, you are on the right track. Here are some suggestions of things to look out for:

- Is the teacher encouraging completion and perfectionism, even in the most subtle ways? Do you notice that this makes you strive to do a more advanced version of a move/posture? Do you tend to override the small quiet voice of your body telling you to stop or slow down?
- Are you encouraged to stay creative, playful, and open-minded? Are you given options that suit your body type/health condition, such as bending your legs in a forward bend instead of keeping them straight? Try to adopt a beginner's mind and sustain your attention throughout the entire movement/training session, making the first move as important and correct as the last, and the small movement as important as the bigger one. Do you feel able to move at your own speed, or do you think you have to fit in with the group?
- By developing your inner observation skills you will naturally create and nurture a nonjudgmental attitude. Wherever you are, that's where you

are and that is perfectly okay. Where you are at present, that is your starting point. Take this attitude toward your body and your eating habits and always start from a kind place.

- As soon as you notice you are pushing yourself too hard, step back, refocus on your breathing, and expand your awareness into the entire body. This will help you to feel that the entire body has to be part of the practice. Is your teacher encouraging you to work with your body in this explorative way, trusting its wisdom?

- By practicing patience and persistence you are taking care of your body: you trust its ability to know when to stop and when to go that bit further. So you are developing awareness, focus, and tuning in, which are important aspects in your effort to change the way you eat.

- Try to keep your eyes closed when you are doing lying down or seated postures. This helps you to turn your awareness inwardly as you do in the body scan, enabling you to connect with the entire body and its depth, and bringing you back in sync with yourself and with others.

Mindful yoga

There are different ways to practice yoga and over the last 100 years the practice has become very much more workout-focused and less mindful. Often classes are taught in gyms. They tend to be drop-in classes where people with very different experience and ability join in together. Even a highly skilled teacher can find this challenging.

This has led to the idea that yoga might not be for the normal person, only for the young and bendy. This might be true as far as some of the newly developed styles of yoga are concerned, but there are lots of yoga practices that are beneficial for every person, of any weight and of any age. The practice of yoga was meant to be for everybody who wants to live a more fulfilling and meaningful life. The word "yoga," after all, means a connection of body, mind, and soul.

In fact, any activity done with a mindful attitude can help you to get through the day with ease, calm, and enough energy to keep going. On top of that you can discover gifts of tranquillity and focus you thought you could never have.

A short yoga practice

- Free up the neck: sit on a chair, looking ahead, then allow the chin to drop on to the breast bone. Then look up again. Repeat a few times and be very mindful of the movement that occurs in your neck/cervical spine. Come back to the start position and feel the neck now.
- Sit upright, look ahead, and allow the head to drop forward onto the chest. Now gently let the head sway left and right in small movements like a pendulum. Follow the movement attentively. When you have repeated it 5–7 times come back to the upright position and feel the neck now.
- Free up the shoulders: you can do this movement sitting, lying down, or even in the morning before you get out of bed. With the arms along the sides of the body, draw the right shoulder up toward the ear and let it sink back to the start position. Repeat several times, then stop and sense into the upper body and shoulder. Then draw the right shoulder forward and back. Repeat several times and come back to the start position. Feel the upper body and shoulder now. Then bring these two movements together and start to circle the right shoulder. When you have finished, compare the right side with the left. Do you notice any difference? In size, temperature, weight, length? Now repeat on the other side and then circle both shoulders together.

Mindful walking

Most of us can engage in a practical exercise such as walking. It is safe, doesn't cost anything and with proper clothing can be done anytime and anywhere. It can be done whether you are old or young, stiff or mobile, healthy and fit, or recovering from illness and exhaustion. Walking can accommodate each one of us, whoever we are, whatever condition we are in. It has many health benefits, as it conditions the heart and lungs, burns calories, helps to destress, and increase vitality by expeling stale air from the lungs. The goal is not to reach any destination but to develop understanding and awareness of the sensations that occur in the body while you are walking.

Become aware of the muscles and the joints in your body as you move. Start with some slow steps and notice how your foot makes contact with the ground. Then pay attention to the lifting of the heel and the push-off from the toes, the weight distribution on your foot, the engagement of your calf muscles and hamstrings, and the ankle, knee, and hip joints. Notice your trunk swaying and your arms swinging. Start to playfully increase your speed, but remember, it is not about reaching any destination: your goal is awareness of the body moving.

Scan your body from head to toes for any unnecessary tension. Be especially aware of the areas around the neck, shoulders, and lower back. Ask yourself what is needed to make this movement light and enjoyable.

Lengthen your stride and as you do so see if your arms can swing a bit further. Try to lead the movement from your pelvis and navel center, rather than from your head or chest.

Walk for at least 10 minutes and then gradually reduce your pace.

After movement

People who participated in our mindful movement sessions spoke about their experiences. Here are some of the insights they shared with us:

- I am less anxious now and have become a more calm and confident person.
- At times I felt I was living a zombie-like existence. Yoga brought me back to a feeling of connectedness with myself and others.
- Through the mindful movements I became aware how much I have lived in my head and ended up worrying about everything. My body can move, even if I am not an athlete.
- Mindful movement helped me to stop splitting my body into parts I like and parts I dislike. I realized the body only functions as a whole.
- The yoga stretches and relaxation have helped me to get in touch with my body and my running has greatly improved.
- Despite my weight I feel comfortable doing these moves as they are simple, they feel safe, and everybody has their eyes closed. No competition! What a relief!
- The movement practices got me back in touch with a joy I had forgotten I knew.

Encourage yourself to engage in a movement practice you really like (how about dancing!?) and it can help you to relieve the stress that has been stored in your body. Mindful movement can bring you a feeling of coming home, to the here and now, through self-acceptance, awareness, and kindness.

Guided Practice: Salmon & Bulghur Wheat Pilaf

After any activity, your energy levels need restoring. Energy comes from carbohydrates and while some of these should be eaten in moderation, plenty of others are extremely healthy and can be eaten as part of a mindful diet. Protein is also essential for healthy, strong muscles, and it helps you to feel full for longer.

The recipes in this section have been chosen to provide you with the right sort of energy and balanced nutrition for an active lifestyle. It is important to balance movement with rest. Your lung capacity improves with exercise. The freeness of breath, exhilaration and release of endorphins produce a fantastic rush, but it is important to take the time to enjoy this as well as to contrast the experience with calm and stillness. Return to slow breathing and find the stillness and peace required for mindful eating.

This first recipe here is quick, easy, and versatile—excellent for those with a busy, active lifestyle. Salmon is great source of protein and essential oils. Its vibrant color is always a delight to look at and as the bright red warms to a delicate pink, you can appreciate every stage of the cooking process. Bulghur wheat is rich in protein and minerals and has a nutty taste. It provides an excellent contrast to the flaky, oily salmon and crisp green vegetables.

As you eat, notice how your body receives the food. Let it reward your movement and restore your energy levels. Remember to eat slowly, returning the body and breath to a state of stillness and peace. It is common for people who have exercised to overeat and treat food as a reward, so remember to pause frequently and really listen to your body's fullness signals.

In particular, the zingy lemon will bring out the light flavor of the salmon. Appreciate how fresh that feels with the green vegetables. Imagine every mouthful is helping to restore your body. Take the time to appreciate how energized and satisfied you feel.

salmon & bulghur wheat pilaf

Calories per serving 478 • Serves 4
Preparation time 10 minutes • Cooking time 10–15 minutes

15 oz **boneless, skinless salmon**
1¾ cups **bulghur wheat**
⅔ cup **frozen peas**
7 oz **string beans**, chopped
2 tablespoons chopped **chives**
2 tablespoons chopped **flat-leaf parsley**
salt and **black pepper**

To serve
2 **lemons**, halved
low-fat yogurt

Cook the salmon in a steamer or microwave for about 10 minutes. Alternatively, wrap it in foil and cook in a preheated oven, 350°F, for 15 minutes.

Meanwhile, cook the bulghur wheat according to the directions on the package and boil the peas and beans. Alternatively, cook the bulghur wheat, peas, and beans in the steamer with the salmon.

Flake the salmon and mix it into the bulghur wheat with the peas and beans. Fold in the chives and parsley and season to taste. Serve immediately with lemon halves and yogurt.

tuna steaks with wasabi dressing

Calories per serving 279 • Serves 4
Preparation time 5 minutes • Cooking time 6–7 minutes

4 **tuna steaks**, about 5 oz each
2 teaspoons **mixed peppercorns**, crushed
8 oz **sugar snap peas**
1 teaspoon **toasted sesame oil**
2 teaspoons **sesame seeds**, lightly toasted

Dressing
2 tablespoons **light soy sauce**
4 tablespoons **mirin**
1 teaspoon **sugar**
1 teaspoon **wasabi paste**

Season the tuna steaks with the crushed peppercorns. Heat a griddle pan over medium-high heat and griddle the tuna steaks for 2 minutes on each side until browned but still pink in the center. Remove from the pan and let rest.

Put the sugar snap peas in a steamer basket and lower into a shallow saucepan of boiling water so that the peas are not quite touching the water. Drizzle with the sesame oil, cover, and steam for 2–3 minutes or until tender. Alternatively, cook the peas in a bamboo or electric steamer.

Place all of the dressing ingredients in a screw-top jar and seal with a tight-fitting lid. Shake vigorously until well combined.

Divide the sugar snap peas between 4 serving dishes, then cut the tuna steaks in half diagonally and arrange over the peas. Drizzle with the prepared dressing and sprinkle with the sesame seeds. Serve immediately, with cellophane rice noodles, if liked.

AWARENESS POINTS
- Cut the tuna into small bite-size flakes and let them melt in your mouth. This recipe is extremely filling if you leave enough time and space between each mouthful.
- Taste a pinprick amount of wasabi paste and note how large and powerful the taste is for something so small.
- Listen to the crisp vegetables and seeds and remind yourself that you are replenishing your body with freshness and energy.

poached eggs & spinach

Calories per serving 291 • Serves 4
Preparation time 5 minutes • Cooking time 8–10 minutes

4 strips of **cherry tomatoes on the vine**, about 6 tomatoes on each
2 tablespoons **balsamic syrup** or **glaze**
1 small bunch of **basil leaves**
1 tablespoon **distilled vinegar**
4 large **eggs**
4 thick slices of **whole-wheat bread**
reduced-fat butter, to spread (optional)
3½ oz **baby spinach leaves**
salt and **black pepper**

Lay the cherry tomato vines in an ovenproof dish, drizzle with the balsamic syrup or glaze, scatter with the basil leaves, and season with salt and pepper. Place in a preheated oven, 350°F, for 8–10 minutes or until the tomatoes begin to collapse.

Meanwhile, bring a large saucepan of water to a gentle simmer, add the vinegar, and stir with a large spoon to create a swirl. Carefully break 2 eggs into the water and cook for 3 minutes. Remove with a slotted spoon and keep warm. Repeat with the remaining eggs.

Toast the whole-wheat bread and butter lightly, if liked.

Heap the spinach onto serving plates and top each plate with a poached egg. Arrange the vine tomatoes on the plates, drizzled with any cooking juices. Serve immediately with the whole-wheat toast, cut into fingers.

AWARENESS POINTS
- This recipe is rich in protein and iron, the perfect breakfast after morning exercise. Take the time to celebrate your work so far and the day ahead.
- Watch the eggs closely during the three minutes they take to poach, noticing every slight movement and change.
- Notice the bright green spinach against the vine red tomatoes and yellow yolk. Can you get all three colors onto your fork for one mouthful?

cashew chicken with peppers

Calories per serving 348 (excluding rice) • Serves 4
Preparation time 10 minutes • Cooking time 15 minutes

2 tablespoons **peanut oil**

1¼ lb **boneless, skinless chicken breasts**, cut into 1 inch pieces

⅓ cup **cashews**

2 **red bell peppers**, cored, seeded, and cut into large pieces

2 **garlic cloves**, chopped

6 **scallions**, halved widthwise and lengthwise

salt

Sauce

1 tablespoon **Chinese rice wine** or **dry sherry**

1 teaspoon **sesame oil**

2 tablespoons **light soy sauce**

½ teaspoon **cornstarch**

4 tablespoons **water**

Combine all the ingredients for the sauce and set the mixture aside.

Heat 1 tablespoon of the peanut oil in a wok over high heat until the oil starts to shimmer. Season the chicken with salt and tip half of it into the wok. Stir-fry for 2–3 minutes until golden, then remove the chicken using a slotted spoon and set aside. Heat the remaining oil and stir-fry the rest of the chicken in the same way. Remove and set aside.

Add the cashews and red bell peppers to the wok and stir-fry for 1 minute. Add the garlic and scallions and cook, stirring, for another minute. Return the chicken to the wok and pour in the sauce. Cook for 3–4 minutes until the chicken is cooked through and the pepper is tender. Serve with rice, if liked.

AWARENESS POINTS

• Taste the sauce and notice the combination of saltiness and sweetness.
• Watch the chicken change color as you stir-fry it in batches. Are all the pieces fully cooked? Do they look similar?
• Notice the size of the portion of rice; make sure it's small. Savor the high-protein chicken. Note the balance of protein on your plate.

fig, bean & toasted pecan salad

Calories per serving 352 • Serves 4
Preparation time 5 minutes, plus cooling • Cooking time 5–6 minutes

⅔ cup **pecans**
7 oz **green beans**, trimmed
4 **fresh figs**, cut into quarters
3½ oz **arugula leaves**
small handful of **mint leaves**
2 oz **Parmesan** or **pecorino cheese**

Dressing
3 tablespoons **walnut oil**
2 teaspoons **sherry vinegar**
1 teaspoon **vincotto** or **balsamic vinegar**
salt and **black pepper**

Heat a heavy-bottomed skillet over medium heat, add the pecans, and dry-fry, stirring frequently, for 3–4 minutes or until browned. Tip onto a small plate and let cool.

Cook the beans in a saucepan of lightly salted boiling water for 2 minutes. Drain, refresh under cold running water, and pat dry with paper towels. Put the beans in a bowl with the figs, pecans, arugula, and mint.

Whisk together all the dressing ingredients in a small bowl and season with salt and black pepper. Pour over the salad and toss well. Shave over the Parmesan or pecorino and serve.

AWARENESS POINTS
• Compare the texture and taste of a pecan before and after frying.
• Explore the crunch of the pecans compared to the fig's softness.
• Imagine your body being cleansed as you eat. Fruit, nuts, and legumes will restore your natural fats and iron levels and are great for your skin.

baked sweet potatoes

Calories per serving 405 • Serves 4
Preparation time 5 minutes • Cooking time 45–50 minutes

4 **sweet potatoes**, about 8 oz
   each, scrubbed
scant 1 cup **sour cream**
2 **scallions**, finely chopped
1 tablespoon chopped **chives**
3½ tablespoons **butter**
salt and **black pepper**

Put the potatoes in a roasting pan and roast in a preheated oven, 425°F, for 45–50 minutes until cooked through.

Combine the sour cream, scallions, chives, and salt and pepper in a bowl.

Cut the baked potatoes in half lengthwise, top with the butter, and spoon over the sour cream mixture. Serve immediately.

AWARENESS POINTS
- Low GI ingredients are good for active diets—think about other dishes for which you can replace normal potatoes with sweet potatoes.
- At what point in the baking time do you notice the appetizing smell? Using your intelligent-body techniques, how hungry do you actually feel?
- Take the time before eating to notice how the bright green specks of scallion pop out of the cream color, and how this looks against the orange sweet potato.

green fruit salad

Calories per serving 167 • Serves 6
Preparation time 15 minutes

10 oz **seedless green grapes**, halved

4 **kiwifruits**, peeled, quartered, and sliced

2 ripe **pears**, peeled, cored, and sliced

4 **passion fruits**, halved

4 tablespoons **concentrated elderflower cordial**

4 tablespoons **water**

1¼ cups **Greek yogurt**

2 tablespoons **clear honey**

Put the grapes, kiwifruits, and pears in a bowl. Using a teaspoon, scoop the seeds from 3 of the passion fruits into the bowl. Mix 2 tablespoons of the cordial with the measurement water and drizzle over the salad. Gently toss together and spoon into 6 glass tumblers.

Stir the remaining undiluted cordial into the yogurt, then mix in the honey. Spoon into the glasses.

Decorate with the remaining passion fruit seeds and serve.

AWARENESS POINTS
- Enjoy the vibrant greens and fresh juice as you chop the fruits.
- Taste a seed from the passion fruit—is it tart or sweet?
- How does the honey contrast with the fresh fruit tastes?

spiced beef & vegetable stew

Calories per serving 325 • Serves 4
Preparation time 15 minutes • Cooking time 2½ hours

1 lb **lean braising** or **stewing steak**

2 tablespoons **canola** or **olive oil**

1 large **onion**, chopped

1 inch piece of **fresh ginger root**, peeled and finely grated

2 **chiles**, sliced

2 **garlic cloves**, crushed

2½ cups **beef stock**

5 **star anise**

1 teaspoon **Chinese five-spice powder**

1 **cinnamon stick**

1 teaspoon **fennel seeds**

2 **dried kaffir lime leaves**

1 **lemon grass stalk**, chopped

1 teaspoon **black peppercorns**

2 tablespoons **shoyu** or **tamari sauce**

13 oz **carrots**, cut into ½ inch slices

1 lb 2 oz **daikon** or **turnips**, cut into ½ inch slices

Chives, to garnish

Cut the steak into 1 inch cubes.

Heat the oil in a wok over medium heat. Add the onion, ginger, and chiles and stir-fry for 5–7 minutes.

Turn the heat up to high, add the beef, and stir-fry for 5–10 minutes until lightly browned.

Add the garlic, stock, star anise, Chinese five-spice powder, cinnamon, fennel seeds, lime leaves, lemon grass, peppercorns, and shoyu or tamari sauce and stir well.

Bring the mixture back to a boil, then reduce the heat, cover the pan, and simmer gently for 1½ hours, stirring occasionally. Add the carrots and daikon or turnips and continue cooking, covered, for another 45 minutes or until the vegetables have softened.

Skim any fat off the surface and garnish with the chives before serving.

AWARENESS POINTS

• Pause to smell each herb and spice before you add it to the stew.

• Apply the same appreciation when eating. Pause after each mouthful to smell the stew again. Can you make out the star anise? And the lemon grass?

• Stews are a great way to load protein and vegetables into your diet. Batch cook this recipe and rest assured you will have a healthy meal to heat up after work whenever you wish.

4 No breath, no life

Isn't it amazing that the most valuable aspect of being alive is hardly ever spoken about—the breath? It seems that we have forgotten to honor and value our breathing, but we can learn to become more conscious of it through the power of awareness.

Breathing is even more important than what we eat and drink. We can live without water or food for several days, but without breath our brain would shut down within minutes. In Los Angeles, "oxygen bars" have been established to help you stay young and beautiful, and of course the managers charge you quite a lot for the provision of an extra dose of oxygen.

How we breathe affects our energy levels, what we do, our relationships, how we move and exercise, and what we eat. And the same is true the other way around—what we do, our relationships, how we move and exercise, and what we eat affects our breathing.

But breathing is not only essential for our physical health. It also helps our minds automatically get into the present moment. It is only in the present moment that we can see and understand our mental state. This is especially important when we eat not because we are hungry, but because we are emotionally upset or just bored.

Our body's wellness and the breath

Our body is made to breathe. Our lungs can expand the upper torso to the front, the back, and the sides. The diaphragm brings movement to the belly and to the back, and when we become attentive, we can feel the breath in our groins, in our shoulder joints, and in our entire body.

In between our first breath and our last, life happens. When we observe our breathing closely, we understand that every moment of our life is mirrored in our breathing—in its depth, its rhythm, its length, and even its speed.

Relaxation, emotions, and the breath

Each and every time we breathe in deeply and slowly, our abdomen expands and starts massaging our organs—liver, kidneys, and stomach. Each time we breathe in through our nostrils, we actually cleanse the air we are breathing of dust particles, and there is less danger of bacteria entering our throat and lungs. This is why most Eastern techniques—yoga and Tai Chi, for example—advise breathing in and out through your nostrils.

Many philosophies, and also modern teachers of exercise, tell you to take a deep breath and relax. This common wisdom is based on a principle known as the Herring/Briar Reflex. When you inhale fully and slowly, you stretch receptors in your lungs, which send signals for relaxation to your cardiovascular system. This triggers a decrease in heart rate. In addition, deep breathing floods your body with oxygen, which is, after all, its primary fuel. It opens your chest and stimulates your heart center, or in energy medicine terminology, the heart chakra. Simply breathing with awareness can calm your mind and nourish your body at any time.

When we feel down and depressed, our breath will be shallow and slow, often with a sighlike quality. When we have eaten too much, we struggle to breathe deeply. After a walk through the woods, we feel refreshed and energized.

By breathing, we bring oxygenated blood to our cells and organs, helping to repair them and helping them to work properly. Our breath is like waves, coming and going, rolling and turning, and like the waves stopping water from getting stagnant, our breathing should dispense with stagnant air. If we breathe in a shallow fashion, we are not emptying our lungs completely and therefore stagnant air remains. No wonder, then, that we feel tired and tend to eat too much to regain our energy.

Past, future, and eating in the now

To learn to be with the present is not for the fainthearted. It takes courage, because it can be painful and frightening when, for example, we have just stuffed down another bout of food. To learn to be present with kind attention, we use the breath. It is always with us, easy to track and accessible, and absolutely free. As the breath occurs *only* in the now, using it is an excellent way to stay present and to remind us to connect with our reality.

It is true for most of us that, for a big part of our lives, we have lived more in the past or in the future than in the present moment. Unfortunately, thinking of the past or the future will make us more stressed and agitated since we can't do anything about either of them in this moment. Hence we tend to look for something to soothe us, often food or drink.

It can be helpful to reflect on past events, so we can gain insight into what we did and why we did it, in case we need to do things differently now. Thinking about doing it differently is happening in the present moment. However, by the time we are doing it differently, it is already taking place in a new present moment (which was the future when we first thought about it). We often tend to be trapped in repetitive, negative, or attached thinking about the past and future. This can trigger a low mood, remembering all the highlights and good times we had (attachment), which alas have gone now and may never return; or it can fill us with regret (another type of low mood) about what we have done wrong or missed doing.

The future is also important, because our aspirations and intentions give us direction. Only when we know what we aspire to can we collect our energies and move toward our goal. But even if we know our goal, the first step and all those that follow happen in the present moment. We can dream, hope, and have wonderful fantasies, but we still have to take one step at a time, and each step is occurring in the present moment. Thinking about the future can also trigger low mood, as we might compare the much more colorful and successful future of what "might be" with the reality of what actually is. Reality often lacks the splendor of our imagination.

Wherever you are at this moment, that's where you are. That is your starting point. The past is gone and the future is not yet here. It is only in this moment that we can make new and healthier choices. It is in this moment that we can start again and decide the direction of our eating life.

Breath therapy

The work of well-known breath and speech therapists, including Ilse Middendorf, Alice Scharschuh, and Elsa Gindler, was later taken up by Western psychologists Wilhelm Reich and Alexander Lowen. They were interested in using the strong link between a balanced body and a healthy mind to heal their patients. By encouraging their clients to breathe differently, they helped them to access strong emotions that had been hidden and stored away. The breath could come to a place of unforced natural flow, which increased the experience of a relaxed body and a relaxed mind.

Before you eat, particularly if you are driven to eat by being upset, turn to your breath. By paying attention to your breath and understanding its patterns, you can make it your ally. In this world, we all feel lonely, rejected, and unanchored at times. Your breath can help you to feel calmed, soothed, and happy. The breath is your anchor to yourself and to a sense of being alive and cared for.

Every single moment in our life presents us with choices. Every moment we can be in touch with what our breathing presents us with—an opportunity to make the right choice. If we want to eat chocolate, we can, but mindfully. We can see how much of the chocolate we want to eat, what triggered the wish to eat it, and how we feel while we are eating it, and afterward. Through this entire experience, we breathe and open up to the understanding of what we do more fully.

Practices

To be in touch with the breath as it is happening right now is a special way of feeling and is not always easy. You are tuning in to the sensations, feelings, and perceptions of what is happening right now as you are breathing in and breathing out. You will notice that what we call breathing is a bundle of different sensations. Over time you will notice that being lost in thought is directly accompanied by a muscular tension in your body, a holding of, and rigidity around, your breath.

Here there are just two simple practices to get in touch with your breathing. It can be difficult to begin with, but with understanding, similar to when you start to eat more mindfully, you will see the quality of your breath changing and with it your wellbeing. Do either of these practices every day and you will learn to tune in and find out what is really needed. Mental awareness will assist you to make the right choices with food.

First, you might notice the pattern of your breathing, shallow or deep, and with it your energy levels; whether it's fast or slow and, with that, your mind's state of agitation or dullness. Slowly, depth, length, and intensity will develop and begin to make a difference to how you feel in your body and mind.

Our bodies know how to breathe. Sometimes when we observe our breathing, it can feel blocked, shorter, or constricted. There is no right or wrong way of breathing. Your breath will change according to the situation you are in. When you judge your breath, it brings trouble. Just notice it. At times, the breath feels deep and shallow and can move freely, and at other times it feels blocked and can be short or long. We are changing all the time, and so is the breath.

If you have a breath-related condition, such as asthma, or any severe allergies, and turning your awareness toward your breath feels uncomfortable and makes you tense, you may wish to skip the next practice. To let go of the tension that surrounds your breath, go easy, and instead of sitting for 10 minutes every day, just notice the moments when your breath opens up and feels free, such as when you sigh, or yawn, or after a good run.

Try to cultivate curiosity about your breathing and experiment with it. Just try this now. It will take only five minutes.

Experimenting with the breath
(This is largely based on breath awareness as taught by Thanissaro Bhikkhu.)

- Sit down comfortably and keep warm.
- Where do you feel the breath right now?
- Is it shallow or deep, long or short, fast or slow?
- Has it got a rhythm? What kind of rhythm would make you feel really good?
- How can you receive the breath in your body, in the lungs, and the belly, that is pleasant, enjoyable, and soothing?
- See what works for you.
- Try to think of the breath flowing through the entire body like waves of energy—in through the toes and up to the head, touching along its way all the nerves, blood vessels, bones.
- While you are feeling the breath flowing like this, are there areas in the body where it feels blocked?
- What helps to unblock these areas? Breathing through them, around them, or straight into them? See what works for you. Play with the breath and discover the impact of the breath on your mind.

- Notice that you are aware of your breath and you are aware of the effect it has on your wellbeing.
- When you have found the breath pattern that gives you a sense of fullness and ease, switch your awareness to the mind and notice that it is now centered and calm.
- Notice that you are aware of your breath and you are aware of the calm mind and now turn to awareness itself.

The more often you try this, the more often you will be able to access a calm and centered mind in your daily life, and also during shopping for food, and the food and eating choices you make.

Free and easy breathing

This practice is very relaxing and is suitable for everyone who wants to get back in touch with relaxed breathing. Remember, getting in touch with your breath means letting go of any need to control. It is a lesson in "undoing our doing" and learning to feel good with yourself.

- Find a quiet place where you will not be disturbed for the next 15 minutes.
- Your last meal should have been at least an hour and a half ago.
- If you can, open your window.
- Do some stretching exercises.
- Lie on your back on a soft blanket or yoga mat and place your left palm on your stomach, elbow comfortably on the floor.
- Place your right hand on your left collarbone and feel your breathing here.
- Place your right hand in your left armpit and feel the breathing here.
- Change sides.
- Now with both hands make soft fists and place them on your sternum/chest bone.
- Place your flat hands on the flanks of your chest, then stomach, and then groins.

Stay in each place for one, two or three minutes and notice the effect the touch of the hands has on your breathing.

Tips

- Bigger portions make us eat more—up to 30 percent. So be clever. Use smaller plates and smaller glasses and increase the volume of your food through extra air and water. Air and water are the cheapest ingredients to bulk up your food without adding a calorie to it. In a research project, one group of people ate fresh fruit and another group drank smoothies made with the same amount of fruit. Those who drank the smoothie felt fuller because it had been stirred for a short while and contained more volume through the air that had been whisked into it.

- Don't finish all the food on your plate. For generations brought up during and after the war, this is anathema. Their parents, quite rightly, cherished food. But in some cultures, hosts stop offering you more food only when you leave some on the plate, signaling that you are full. Practice not clearing your plate and it will help you to develop the self-control you need to stop overeating, and help you to eat less.

Guided Practice: Fruity Summer Smoothie

Smoothies are a great way to consume food mindfully. They rely on nutritious ingredients, such as fruit and milk or live yogurt, which nourish our bodies and provide healthy energy. They can include honey for sweetness, or avocado for savory creaminess, and it's easy to vary the recipe to omit dairy products if you prefer. Whisked to provide an airy lightness, smoothies can be sipped and savored, and are filling without being heavy.

We breathe deeply when we smell something pleasant. As you begin to make this smoothie, savor the delicious aroma of the sweet berries as you prepare them. Enjoy the heady scent of ripe peaches as you cut into them and release their juice. How does the skin feel to touch? When you chop fruit, or use a noisy blender to mix the ingredients or crush ice, do you hold your breath?

Notice your breathing, and try to keep it slow and mindful. Appreciate the anticipation of the exotic flavor combinations, and choose a suitable glass to display the bright color of this energy-providing power drink.

How will you drink it? Will you sip it through a straw? Perhaps you could sit outside and enjoy the fresh air, if the weather is good enough.

It can be hard to drink mindfully, especially when you are thirsty. Being dehydrated can lead to consuming your meals much too fast, which in turn leads to overindulgence. Drink a large glass of water before you begin, to rehydrate your body and allow yourself to tune in to what your body requires.

Remember to savor the smell of the fruit as you begin to drink the smoothie. Notice the creaminess, the sharp tang of the fruit, the sweetness, and the pleasant chill from the ice. Were you too hot when you started drinking it? Can you feel the cool sensation traveling through your chest, refreshing your body? Pause, and breathe deeply and mindfully between each mouthful.

Although blended, a smoothie is still nourishing, satisfying food, and it is important to notice when your stomach is full. When you have finished, return to the breath, and to stillness.

fruity summer smoothie

Calories per serving 103 • Makes 4 x 10 oz glasses
Preparation time 2 minutes

2 **peaches**, halved, pitted, and
  chopped
2 cups **strawberries**, hulled
scant 2½ cups **raspberries**
1¾ cups **skim** or **lowfat milk**
ice cubes

Put the peaches in a blender or food
processor with the strawberries and
raspberries and blend to a smooth puree,
scraping the mixture down from the sides
of the bowl if necessary.

Add the milk and blend the ingredients
again until the mixture is smooth and
frothy. Pour the milkshake over the ice
cubes in tall glasses.

miso chicken broth

Calories per serving 163 • Serves 4
Preparation time 10 minutes • Cooking time 20 minutes

1 tablespoon **sunflower oil**

2 **boneless, skinless chicken breasts**, diced

8 oz **cup mushrooms**, sliced

1 **carrot**, cut into thin sticks

¾ inch piece of **fresh ginger root**, peeled and grated

2 large pinches of **crushed dried red pepper flakes**

2 tablespoons **brown rice miso paste**

4 tablespoons **mirin** or **dry sherry**

2 tablespoons **light soy sauce**

5 cups **water**

2 **bok choy**, thinly sliced

4 **scallions**, thinly sliced

4 tablespoons chopped **fresh cilantro**

Heat the oil in a saucepan, add the chicken, and fry for 4–5 minutes, stirring until golden. Add the mushrooms and carrot sticks, then the ginger, chiles, miso, mirin or sherry, and soy sauce.

Pour in the measurement water and bring to a boil, stirring, then simmer for 10 minutes.

Add the bok choy, scallions, and chopped cilantro and cook for 2–3 minutes until the bok choy has just wilted. Ladle into bowls and serve.

AWARENESS POINTS
- Perform a three-minute breathing exercise while you allow the soup to cool.
- Before you begin to eat, take three long breaths, focusing in turn on the ginger, soy, and cilantro.
- Pause after each spoonful. Try putting your spoon down on the table after each swallow, then pick it up and go back for more.

steamed citrus sea bass

Calories per serving 256 • Serves 4
Preparation time 15 minutes • Cooking time 20 minutes

1 whole **sea bream** or sea **bass**, about 1 lb 10 oz–2 lb, scaled and cleaned
¼ cup **chicken stock** or **water**
¼ cup **Chinese rice wine** or **dry sherry**
rind of 1 small **orange**, thinly sliced
1 inch piece of **fresh ginger root**, peeled and thinly sliced
1 teaspoon **superfine sugar**
3 tablespoons **light soy sauce**
½ teaspoon **sesame oil**
1 **garlic clove**, thinly sliced
3 **scallions**, thinly sliced
1 tablespoon **peanut oil**

Score 3 diagonal slits along each side of the fish with a sharp knife, then repeat in the opposite direction.

Cut 2 large pieces of foil about 1½ times the length of the fish. Place the fish in the center of the double layer of foil and lift it up around the fish slightly. Pour the stock and rice wine over the fish, then scatter with the orange rind and half the ginger.

Place a circular rack inside a wok and pour in enough water to come just below the top of the rack. Place the lid on the wok and bring the water to a rolling boil. Carefully sit the open fish parcel on the rack, cover with the lid, and steam for 15–18 minutes until the flesh inside the slits is opaque. Carefully remove the fish from the wok and place on a serving dish.

Stir together the sugar, soy sauce, and sesame oil, then pour over the fish with the garlic, scallions, and remaining ginger.

Heat the peanut oil in a small skillet over high heat until smoking hot, then pour it over the fish to crisp up the scallions and ginger. Serve immediately.

AWARENESS POINTS
• Think of wrapping the fish as a ritual, and every ingredient as a special part of the parcel.
• As the fish steams, breathe slowly and absorb the aromas.
• Notice how the peanut oil releases and heightens the smell of the ginger and scallions.

citrus refresher

calories per serving 274 • Serves 4

Preparation time 10 minutes, plus cooling • Cooking time 6–7 minutes

⅔ cup chilled **orange juice**
from a carton
⅔ cup **water**
⅔ cup **superfine sugar**
juice of ½ **lemon**
2 **ruby grapefruit**
4 **oranges** (a mix of ordinary
and **blood oranges**, if
available)
1 **orange-fleshed melon**
½ **pomegranate**

Pour the orange juice and measurement water into a saucepan, add the sugar, and heat gently until the sugar has dissolved, then simmer for 5 minutes until syrupy. Remove the pan from the heat and mix in the lemon juice.

Cut a slice off the top and bottom of each grapefruit, then cut away the rest of the peel in downward slices using a small serrated knife. Holding the fruit over a bowl, cut between the membranes to release the segments. Cut a slice off the top and bottom of the oranges, then cut away the rest of the peel. Cut into segments and add to the bowl.

Cut the melon in half, scoop out the seeds, then cut away the peel and dice the flesh. Add to the citrus fruit, then pour over the cooled syrup. Flex the pomegranate to release the seeds, sprinkle over the salad, then chill until ready to serve.

AWARENESS POINTS
• Think of this as a palette cleanser; imagine it renewing all your senses in the now moment.
• If you can find blood oranges, how do they compare in bitterness and sweetness to the grapefruit and ordinary oranges?
• As you flex the pomegranate, listen to the sound of the skin breaking and focus on every tiny, beautiful seed.

5 Destination guilt food— how to deal with cravings

This book is based on the premise that behind every weight problem is a human being. Most of us have dieted or have seen friends losing and gaining weight. Most diets don't work because they deal with food intake only, not with the human being who consumes it. We gain weight because we eat when we are not hungry; we become too thin when we deprive ourselves of food when we do need it. In both cases, the mind overrides simple body symptoms and tries to solve unpleasant moods and feelings by eating, or not eating.

We look for solutions to our inner dissatisfaction by seeking satisfying experiences through food. Unfortunately, this won't work. We can get satisfaction through food when we are hungry, but we can't feed the longings of our mind with food.

We have to learn to differentiate between the needs of our body and the needs and desires of our mind and soul.

Important needs

What are human beings' important needs? To answer this, we can consult American pyschologist Abraham Maslow's (1908–70) hierarchy of needs. He systemized and organized our needs into a pyramid. According to his model, our physiological needs must be mostly satisfied before the individual can start to deal with safety and security needs. Once we feel safe and secure, love and belonging needs can emerge and be given more attention. From a safe place of belonging and shelter, we develop self-esteem/acceptance and from this we can grow to address self-actualizing needs.

Once the basic needs have been met, we have to face more challenging territory—our wanting mind. It is the desiring mind that whispers to us and makes us eat this, buy that, wear this, choose that. Sometimes the desiring voice is quite gentle. It might even give us the freedom to choose to eat or not, depending on the situation. Other times, you might feel you are in the grip of something so powerful that you can't resist: "I want it, and I want it now." When that happens and we feel we aren't being given a choice, no clear decision-making process kicks in. We are on autopilot. It doesn't matter if our desires are good or harmful, we blindly follow them.

Try this experiment. Wait until you are hungry before going to the supermarket or grocery store, and observe your shopping behavior. You will end up putting much more food into your cart or basket than you planned. Everything will look so appetizing and you may even decide to make a dessert for later. Next time, go shopping when you're not hungry. How do things differ?

The hungry ghost

An image that mindfulness-course participants find most helpful is that of the "hungry ghost." They can immediately relate to it. Hungry ghosts are depicted as large mystical beings with huge, expanded bellies and narrow throats. They eat all day, but their narrow throats prevent them from swallowing enough food to make them feel full. No matter how much they eat, they feel empty, unhappy, and deprived.

The hungry ghost has been with us for a very long time. For example, when we were children, we had three choices of ice-cream flavors— chocolate, vanilla, and strawberry. When more flavors became available, we wanted even more. We added chocolate sprinkles and were still not content. Then came the cream and the little umbrella and still we were not happy. That is the nature of the hungry ghost—never satisfied, always whispering to us and persuading us to go for something more, which will supposedly bring us happiness and rarely ever does.

It's not just food. The hungry ghost can present itself in feelings of being deprived of all the pleasures of life that others enjoy. The others have richer parents, nicer brothers and sisters, a better figure, sunnier and more exciting vacations, newer cars, bigger TV screens, and they can eat in the most expensive restaurants. They seem to have all the objects and experiences you don't have. Your assumption may be that they are the happy ones and you crave their happiness.

The hungry ghost lives in all of us. Body-centered therapy (see Chapter 2 "The intelligent body") describes the oral phase of childhood development, dealing with a newborn baby's need to be fed, warm, and cared for. If this stage of natural development is deficient, we grow up with the belief that this world will not nourish us. We feel hungry for food, love, and attention.

To help you understand the presence of the hungry ghost, you need to be aware of it, get to know it, learn its language: "I have to eat this cookie; I need to buy this drink; I love this pizza, this restaurant, this special type of bread; I hate carbohydrates; I want to buy this food processor so I can make those magic juices; I hate parties where there is a lot of food; I don't want a carrot stick instead of potato chips; I want more exercise, less chocolates, and I want to look beautiful and gorgeous and then I will be happy and loved."

The hungry ghost does not always talk that loudly. It can convince you with murmurs—"Just this first chocolate praline, ice cream or ..." Its whispers make us forget that even the most delicious food can make us feel sick when we have too much of it or when it does not agree with us. "Just one more spoonful of this delicious meal" and we forget that soon afterward we'll feel the tightness of a bulging stomach, and the tiredness from having eaten too much. The ghost's voice is so gentle and persuasive that we forget how we felt last time we gave in to it. Furthermore, we have forgotten to notice our body's sensations/cues, which have told us already, some time ago, that we have had enough.

Try writing down, and so externalizing, your ghost's attempts to make you act obediently.

- Describe how it influences you. Is it lonely, empty, powerless, manipulative, or desperate?
- What does it want you to do? Buy the new gadget, pair of shoes, diet book, magic powder, or weight-loss program? What does it want you to become? The best cook in the world, the wine connoisseur, or the person who always knows the latest trend in food shopping? What does it want you to own? The magic soup/bread/hotch-potch maker? What does it want you to get rid of? The flabby belly, the big thighs?
- When does it shout the most? During office hours, with the cookie tin near the coffee machine? On your way home when you walk past a wonderful bakery? On vacation when you are relaxed? With your friends on a night out? When you are desperate anyway? Try to learn its pattern of behavior.

You will notice that the hungry ghost makes you eat and shop, but the action of doing so is almost always triggered by a deep feeling of suffering and emotional hunger. Our wish to change our weight is often linked to these underlying emotions.

To understand our hungry ghost, we have to befriend it in an act of self-compassion. We do this by learning to become more closely attentive to our strongest feelings and desires. In order to deal with our cravings, we have to relate to our intense feelings rather than pretending they are not there. We have to face them without acting them out and without repressing them.

In mindful eating, you are invited to become close to your strong feelings and to connect with your own vulnerability, gentleness, and compassion. You are asked to let go of hate, and by doing so, heal the hurt that initially created the pattern of eating when you feel emotionally upset.

By befriending your hungry ghost, you can start looking for the nourishment that is of a different kind from food—nourishment for the mind and heart. It opens up the possibility of freedom from cravings, and from there new choices become available.

Next time you experience a craving, ask yourself the following questions, and write down the answers:

- Am I really hungry? How do I know?
- Is my body hungry, like the wolf that leaves the safety of the forest because it is starving? Is it food I need or might a hot bath, a walk, a swim, or a gentle touch do instead?
- In case my body is hungry, what does it need right now?
- Is my mind hungry? For music, to read a book, conversation?
- Is my heart hungry? Do I need to belong and feel loved? Do I need to meet a friend who listens? Do I need support to deal with challenges at work? Do I need assistance from a family member?

Hungry ghost v. austerity master

The hungry ghost has a sibling, the austerity master, and he is at his happiest when you are depriving yourself of even the smallest pleasure. Instead of giving in to the demands and never-ending desires of the hungry ghost, you won't have any sugar, because "sugar is bad for you." The people who are in the grip of the austerity master never stop telling you how bad all the stuff is that you are eating. But don't be fooled. In most cases, the desire for sugar has just gone underground.

It is important to understand that the hungry ghost and the austerity master are two sides of the same coin. The more you rely on your willpower, the more the craving will persist. "What you resist will persist." When you suppress your need for food, you will keep thinking about it, become obsessed with it. When is the next meal? How can I avoid it?

The big solution

Mindful eating is not about turning away from what we are doing but turning toward it and becoming more aware of it. If you practice any or all of the exercises in this book, you will open the door of insight and learn to notice the triggers that unleash your cravings. As we become more mindful, we pursue only those that we see as beneficial and let go of those that harm us and others.

We all have different strategies to help us attain this goal of feeling happy and fulfilled. For some it can be the purchase of a new gadget, finding the right partner, buying a special cake, a blissful experience during meditation, or the feeling of flow during an evening run when all work is done. It may also be getting rid of an old phone, throwing away the boyfriend's sweater, replacing the old car with a new one ... the examples are manifold. You may think that the next thing that comes along will bring you the happiness we all want so much for our lives.

All these strategies follow a similar pattern:

- You feel that something is lacking, missing in your life.
- You identify the cause for this feeling.
- You think about a solution to this problem.

Yet every desire has a different solution and reaches for a different type of satisfaction. Although it may be wonderful to have these aspirations, it is paramount to deal with them skillfully, and now we are coming to the nub of understanding our cravings.

One desire surpasses all others and that is the wish to experience joy, happiness that is independent of external factors. This desire is born out of our wish to feel loved once again, at ease and at home in this world, as we did in the womb or sometimes still when we were little ones. It can be met only when you nourish that part of you that is hungry beyond anything that you can purchase in a supermarket. This is what we call "skillful desire" and meeting it is the big solution.

Practice—the flesh is willing ... what are your food triggers?

The point of this exercise is to become more aware of what happens just prior to indulging in food or drink, to help you spot the most irresistible triggers.

- Begin by putting your hand on your heart or solar plexus and visualizing being cradled by overflowing compassion. You may want to see somebody who symbolizes kindness for you.
- Review how your overeating or undereating has harmed you and others, and think about how you would like to change this destructive pattern.
- Help your mind to slow down and relax by bringing awareness to your breathing for a little while.
- Fill your mind with care and compassion, and the will to transform your behavior. Allow yourself to be nurtured by this energy.
- Then shift your memory to the last time you overindulged in food. Recall the moment it started, and then go back an instant to when you were just about to start engaging in your addictive behavior. Contemplate what was occurring during that moment. Find out what this starting point feels like.
- Try to bring vivid awareness to your surroundings at that time. Imagine this is all happening right now. Can you see yourself and where you are? Are there any people nearby or are you alone? What odors are present? What tastes do you notice in your mouth and what sounds can you hear? Is your body sensitive or numb? Are you physically and mentally comfortable or uncomfortable?

Any of these factors could be an external trigger. View it with composure and slight detachment, as you would look at a photograph or as if you were a CCTV camera just filming but not reacting to what is recorded.

- Carry on deepening your awareness of what was occurring at that time. Were you in any pain? Did you feel stressed? Were you trying to calm down? Had you just been involved in an argument? Did you feel lonesome? Had someone upset you or had you frustrated yourself? Were you trying to impress anyone? Did life feel disappointing? Was it difficult to cope?

  Any of these could have been internal triggers. View them peacefully and with kindness. Remain aware of that moment as long as you possibly can. Pinpoint those factors that set you off. Accept that this is your current reality, and is the way in which you cope with difficulties for now.

Allow yourself to remain in the realm of compassion and benevolence from which you looked at all the triggers. Visualize this energy being absorbed into your body and healing all the damage, pain, and sickness. Allow your body to experience tranquillity and peace. Imagine the energy of pure kind-hearted wisdom being absorbed into every part of your mind, healing all pessimistic emotions and leaving your mind serene and calm. Rest in this state for as long as you feel you want to, or need to.

Take pleasure in what you have achieved in this meditation, even if aspects of what you remembered were painful, and practice it frequently if you want to get better. In this way you will gain more insight into the triggers that make you eat even when you are not hungry. As you become more aware of the moments before you fall into your unhelpful eating pattern, you will find it easier to change it. You will slowly unlock the origin of dissatisfaction and hurt that is keeping these thinking and behavior patterns in place. Having done this, you can start to find other ways— developing new neuro pathways—of dealing with unhappiness and pain.

A week without

Try giving up any one of the following for a week, and explore the experience:

- sugar
- snacks
- your favorite caffeine
- dairy food
- white flour
- alcohol
- meat
- pre-packed food
- complaining
- internet
- cell phone
- car

Guided Practice: Chocolate Florentines:

Everything in moderation. There are many ways to celebrate food and the act of having something to eat as a reward can be interpreted with a more mindful approach. For example, rather than assuming an unhealthy chocolate cake will boost your mood or transform your stressful day, stop and think about what you actually need. Be true to your body's signals and sensations. It may be that you need to drink more water or boost low blood sugar. In this book, there is no suggestion of giving up your favorite foods and indulgences; simply widen your perception when it comes to treating yourself with food. Is there a healthier alternative? Can you give up caffeine for a week and explore the experience? And when you do treat yourself with food, are you getting the most out of it—savoring every taste sensation rather than eating on autopilot?

The first recipe here, for Chocolate Florentines, is a perfect example of eating something very decadent and delicious in moderation. One Florentine is crammed with textures and flavors to enjoy—slivered almonds, candied peel, rich dark chocolate. One tiny Florentine can contain a wealth of treats. The trick, of course, is to be mindful and not eat the whole lot!

When you add the dried ingredients, one by one, into the melted sugar and butter mixture, notice how different and wonderful they are—a cascade of roughly chopped candied cherries, tumbling hazelnuts, small crystals of candied peel. There are hundreds of combinations of dried fruit and nuts to try.

As you spoon the mixture carefully onto the baking sheets, listen to the crackling of paper and notice the stickiness.

Notice the texture of the thin layer of precious, rich, dark chocolate as you spread it on the Florentines.

Finally, when you come to eat your compact treat, notice the different sweet tastes and textures with every nibble—the sharpness of the candied peel, the smooth, sweet but bitter chocolate, and the crunchy almond slivers. See if you can make a list of 10–20 different sensations. Read it back to yourself and see how one treat can be enhanced with a complex, mindful approach.

chocolate florentines

Calories per serving 126 • Makes 26
Preparation time 30 minutes, plus cooling • Cooking time 20–25 minutes

7 tablespoons **butter**
½ cup **superfine sugar**
3 oz **multicolored candied cherries**, roughly chopped
scant 1 cup **slivered almonds**
2 oz whole **candied peel**, finely chopped
⅓ cup **hazelnuts**, roughly chopped
2 tablespoons **all-purpose flour**
5 oz **semisweet chocolate**, broken into pieces

Put the butter and sugar in a saucepan and heat gently until the butter has melted and the sugar dissolved. Remove the pan from the heat and stir in all the remaining ingredients except the chocolate.

Spoon tablespoons of the mixture, well spaced apart, onto 3 baking sheets lined with nonstick baking parchment. Flatten the mounds slightly. Place 1 baking sheet at a time in the center of a preheated oven, 350°F, and cook for 5–7 minutes until the nuts are golden.

Remove each baking sheet from the oven, then neaten and shape the cooked cookies by placing a slightly larger plain round cookie cutter over the top and rotating to smooth and tidy up the edges. Let cool on the sheets.

Melt the chocolate in a heatproof bowl set over a saucepan of gently simmering water. Peel the cookies off the lining paper and arrange upside down on a wire rack. Spoon the melted chocolate over the flat underside of the cookies and spread the surfaces level. Let cool and harden.

warm chocolate fromage frais

Calories per serving 327 • Serves 6
Preparation time 1 minute • Cooking time 4 minutes

10 oz **semisweet chocolate**, broken into pieces
scant 2¼ cups **fat-free fromage frais**
1 teaspoon **vanilla extract**

Melt the chocolate in a heatproof bowl set over a saucepan of gently simmering water, then remove from the heat.

Add the fromage frais and vanilla extract and quickly stir together.

Divide the chocolate fromage frais among 6 little pots or glasses and serve immediately.

AWARENESS POINTS
• Do you find the warm vanilla smell comforting?
• Notice the silky, thick texture of the melting chocolate as you stir.
• Let each mouthful melt on your tongue, and become aware of each sensation as it arrives.

balsamic strawberries & mango

Calories per serving 100 • Serves 4
Preparation time 5 minutes, plus overnight chilling and standing

3½ cups **strawberries**, hulled
and thickly sliced
1 large **mango**, peeled,
seeded, and sliced
1–2 tablespoons **superfine
sugar**, to taste
3 tablespoons **balsamic
vinegar**
2 tablespoons chopped **mint
leaves**, to decorate

Mix together the strawberries and mango in a large, shallow bowl, sprinkle with the sugar, according to taste, and pour over the balsamic vinegar. Cover with plastic wrap and chill overnight.

Remove the fruit from the refrigerator and let stand for at least 1 hour before serving.

Spoon the fruit into 4 serving bowls, drizzle over the syrup, and serve, sprinkled with the mint.

AWARENESS POINTS
• Mix the freshly cut fruit gently in the bowl with your hands and notice the contrasting textures.
• Notice the colors and the smells of the fruit, sugar, and vinegar before you cover the bowl. When you take it out of the refrigerator, how have the colors changed? Have the aromas combined overnight?
• Taste the fresh mint. How does it change the flavor of the fruit and syrup?

passion fruit panna cotta

Calories per serving 127 • Serves 4
Preparation time 15 minutes, plus cooling and chilling
Cooking time 5 minutes

2 gelatin leaves
8 passion fruit
scant 1 cup half-fat crème
  fraîche
½ cup fat-free Greek yogurt
scant ½ cup water
1 teaspoon superfine sugar
vanilla bean, split

Soften the gelatin leaves in cold water. Halve the passion fruit and remove the seeds, working over a bowl to catch as much juice as you can. Set the seeds faside or decoration.

Combine the crème fraîche, yogurt, and passion fruit juice.

Put the measurement water in a small saucepan, add the sugar and the seeds from the vanilla bean, and heat gently, stirring until the sugar has dissolved. Drain the gelatin and add to the pan. Stir until dissolved, then let cool to room temperature.

Mix the gelatin mixture into the crème fraîche, then pour into 4 ramekins or molds. Chill for 6 hours or until set.

Turn the panna cotta out of their molds by briefly immersing each ramekin in very hot water. Spoon over the reserved seeds to decorate.

AWARENESS POINTS
- Take time to enjoy the sensations of preparing the passion fruit. How does the juice smell and the seeds feel?
- As you mix, heat and combine the ingredients, notice how they change in both texture and color. Remember that you are creating something new.
- Eat the panna cotta slowly, a small mouthful at a time. Mark the intense flavor of the seeds.

st. clement's cheesecake

Calories per serving 245 • Serves 10
Preparation time 10 minutes, plus cooling and chilling
Cooking time 50 minutes

3½ tablespoons **unsalted butter**, plus extra for greasing
6 oz **low-fat oat cookies**, crushed
2 x 8 oz tubs **quark**
⅔ cup **superfine sugar**
2 **eggs**
grated rind and juice of 2 **oranges**
grated rind and juice of 1 **lemon**
scant ½ cup **golden raisins**
juliennes of **orange** and **lemon** rind, to decorate

Lightly grease an 8 inch nonstick, loose-bottomed round cake pan.

Melt the butter in a saucepan, stir in the cookie crumbs, then press them over the bottom and sides of the prepared cake pan. Bake in a preheated oven 300°F, for 10 minutes.

Beat together the remaining ingredients in a bowl, spoon the mixture into the cake pan, and bake for 40 minutes until just firm. Turn off the oven and let the cheesecake cool in the oven for 1 hour.

Transfer the cheesecake to the refrigerator for 2 hours, then serve decorated with juliennes of orange and lemon rind.

AWARENESS POINTS
- Smell the warm butter and cookies as they combine. What feelings or memories does that smell conjure up for you?
- Use the surface of the cheesecake as a blank canvas and decorate any way you please.
- Share the cheesecake with friends or family—notice how it feels to provide your loved ones with a dish you have made yourself.

toffee & chocolate popcorn

Calories per serving 282 • Serves 12
Preparation time 1 minute • Cooking time 4 minutes

4¼ oz **popping corn**
18 tablespoons (2¼ sticks)
  butter
generous 1 packed cup **light
  brown sugar**
2 tablespoons **unsweetened
  cocoa**

Microwave the popping corn in a large bowl with a lid on high (900 watts) for 4 minutes.

Alternatively, cook in a pan with a lid on the stove, on medium heat, for a few minutes until popping.

Meanwhile, gently heat the butter, brown sugar, and cocoa in a pan until the sugar has dissolved and the butter has melted.

Stir the warm popcorn into the mixture and serve.

AWARENESS POINTS
• Listen to the sound of the corn popping against the side of the pan, and be aware of the timing between pops, so that the popcorn does not burn.
• What memories do you have of popcorn? Does it make you think of movie theater seats, or the fairground?
• Think about how to serve the popcorn—perhaps some colorful paper bags would make cheerful containers.

french macarons

Calories per serving 46 • Makes 24
Preparation time 20 minutes, plus standing • Cooking time 10 minutes

butter, for greasing
scant ½ cup **confectioners'**
  sugar
¾ cup **ground almonds**
2 **egg whites**
½ cup **superfine sugar**
pink and **green food coloring**

Grease 2 baking sheets and line with nonstick baking parchment.

Place the confectioners' sugar in a food processor with the ground almonds and blend until fine.

Put the egg whites in a thoroughly clean bowl and whisk until stiff peaks. Gradually whisk in the superfine sugar, whisking well after each addition, until thick and very glossy. Divide the mixture equally between 2 bowls and add a few drops of food coloring to each bowl. Divide the almond mixture between the 2 bowls and stir the mixtures to combine.

Place 1 color in a pastry bag fitted with a ½ inch plain tip and pipe 12 x 1¼ inch circles onto 1 baking sheet. Tap the sheet firmly to smooth the surfaces of the macarons. In a second pastry bag pipe 12 circles in the second color onto the other baking sheet. Let stand for 30 minutes.

Bake in a preheated oven, 325°F, for about 15 minutes, or until the surfaces feel crisp. Let cool before carefully peeling away the paper.

AWARENESS POINTS
• Immerse yourself in the process of transforming the egg whites from their translucent liquid state into bright, stiff, white peaks.
• What food coloring will you use? Have you chosen your favorites, or colors for someone else?
• How does the crisp macaron surface feel when baked? What sound does it make when you peel it from the paper?

frozen fruity yogurt

Calories per serving 194 • Serves 4
Preparation time 15 minutes, plus freezing

scant 2½ cups **fresh** or **frozen raspberries**

3 **nectarines**, skinned, pitted, and chopped

2 tablespoons **confectioners' sugar**

1¾ cups **Greek yogurt**

scant 1 cup **low-fat Greek yogurt**

Put half the raspberries and nectarines in a food processor or blender and process until smooth.

Stir the puree and the rest of the fruit into the remaining ingredients, then transfer to a freezerproof container and freeze for 1 hour. Stir well, then return to the freezer and freeze until solid.

Serve the frozen yogurt in scoops, as you would ice cream. It will keep for up to 1 month in the freezer.

AWARENESS POINTS

• Is your fruit fresh or frozen? Did you choose it at the market, and do you know where it was grown?

• When you blend half the fruit, notice how the combined smell and color is different from those of the separate ingredients.

• Perhaps you could serve this treat in sundae glasses, with long spoons and some sprinkles or chopped nuts, like an ice-cream sundae.

6 Now a thought on nutrition ...

Food journal

Keeping a food diary or journal is a very important part of a mindful eating plan. Leave plenty of space to write about nutrition and allow time for planning. In the beginning it will help to timetable specific periods each day for purchasing, preparing, and eventually enjoying meals and snacks.

On page 103 you'll find a template of things to record each day. It's not just a matter of keeping a note of what you eat; it's important also to remember the tips and practices given throughout this book and to note the sensations you feel when you cook and eat. You can look back and check which items you could replace with healthier alternatives. How often could you replace that tea or coffee with a glass of water?

Record what you ate as soon as possible after eating. Remember it can take at least 20 minutes before you start to feel full. Then note what you were doing before, during, and after eating that item or meal. Then what you felt before, during, and after. Be honest—nobody but you is going to read your journal. As you progress, note your own "awareness points" for recipes, cooking, and eating. Keep a record of the sensations you experienced. When you return to a recipe or eat that foodstuff again, have the feelings and sensations changed?

Look for patterns. What foods affect your moods? What meals leave you feeling happiest and most satisfied? What triggers make you overeat? Try to use this data to plan effectively if you know you will be particularly busy one day or at home, bored, and looking to snack another. What foods give you a negative physical effect such as bloating or tiredness? You may want to track your actual weight or your budget as you go along to see how you are improving or saving.

Food diary tips

- Choose a notebook you like, or use an app if you prefer.
- Be honest.
- Be specific: break complicated foods down by ingredient, size, and/or portion.
- Include snacks and drinks.
- Stick in recipes that you particularly love.
- Read back over your journal and see how your moods and feelings have changed.

DATE | TIME

A brief description of what I ate:

....

How many of an item/what size of portion?

....

Was eating linked to a specific mealtime?

....

Where?

....

Alone or with whom?

....

Activity before, during, and after:

....

Mood before, during, and after:

....

Awareness points:

....

Next time I ate this, the following was different:

....

Basic nutrition

Many people feel burned out and tired, with no energy to spare for living and enjoying.

In order to overcome this state of depletion they often use stimulants to help them wake up and later in the day take relaxants or whatever they perceive as relaxing in order to calm down.

Typical culprits are coffee, energy drinks, and coca cola, chocolate, etc. to boost low energy levels and then smoking or alcohol to release tension. Because most of us are under so much time pressure, we also tend to eat lots of fast foods, which not only contain the wrong kind of fat but also are often overcooked and stored far too long and hence lack many important nutrients, minerals, and vitamins.

So how can we overcome these "quick fixes" and reintroduce into our daily lives a healthier way of eating and fueling "this vehicle that we're driving"?

Nutritionists recommend leaving out refined foods such as white bread, cookies, or fries because they affect blood-sugar levels, often giving a quick high but afterward leaving us more depleted, more tired, and more irritable. Instead, we should be eating more complex carbohydrates, like wholegrain bread and cereals, whole-wheat pasta, vegetables, and beans, because they help us maintain a constant level of energy. Choose foods that are high in vitamins and minerals and have been stored well. Often vegetables that were frozen immediately after harvesting are higher in vitamins than fresh ones that have been on display for days or even weeks.

In order to calm our nerves it is very important to eat oily fish, such as salmon, mackerel, and sardines, or brazil nuts, almonds, or hazelnuts. Similarly, seeds such as pumpkin seeds, sesame seeds, and sunflower seeds will provide us with essential fatty acids, which are vital to maintaining a healthy nervous system.

Another thing that really increases your feeling of wellbeing is drinking enough water. In some research programs, schoolchildren had a bottle of water put on their desks, encouraging them to drink regularly. Their teachers also drank plenty of water and encouraged the children to follow their example. It was found that the children who drank enough water had higher concentration levels and were less aggressive. So it is really important to consume at least 8½ cups of water a day, in order to keep your metabolic rate up and avoid dehydration. Some of the liquid you need is, however, already contained in the fruit and vegetables you eat.

Water facts

- Don't forget, every time you drink coffee or tea you are reducing the amount of water in your body because caffeine has a diuretic effect.
- When you are dehydrated you may experience headaches. You may also suffer from overarousal at night. Hence you are less able to deal with stress. So drink plenty of water and eat lots of fruit and vegetables, as these will introduce extra healthy liquid into your body.
- Vegetables contain at least 75 percent water; some, such as cucumber or watermelon, more like 90 percent. Fruit and vegetables will provide you with vitamins to fight off infection, and minerals to balance the body's metabolism and energy production. Fiber from the fruit and vegetables will help you to eliminate toxins, while complex carbohydrates—that means wholegrain products—will help balance your blood-sugar levels.
- Also remember that thirst is often interpreted as hunger. Before you eat, drink a glass of water and then see how hungry you really are.

Breaking the fast

Should you be pushed for time in the morning or find it difficult to be creative while still trying to get going, it may be helpful prepare muesli in the evening and keep it in the refrigerator. Buy individual types of grain flakes (oats, rice, rye, etc.) and a mixture of nuts, dried fruit, and seeds. If you want to add fresh fruit, you can do this in the morning, although blueberries can be added the night before. Not only are they a powerful antioxidant, they also don't get soggy overnight. In order to soak your muesli, experiment with water, fruit juice, rice, almond, or soy milk or yogurt.

During the colder months you may prefer oatmeal. Once again you can speed up the process by soaking the oats in water overnight: this greatly reduces the cooking time and thus extends the time for mindful eating and digesting. Vary your oatmeal by adding golden raisins, seeds, and spices like cardamom or cinnamon and honey instead of sugar.

Another healthy option for the morning or a daytime snack is a smoothie. If you invest in a juicer you can produce a fabulous concoction in less than five minutes.

Lunch

A wonderful way to enjoy lunch, and somewhat more intriguing than a sandwich, is to prepare soups and stews. Cook several portions at a time and freeze whatever you don't need for future use. Follow the recipes below or create your own. You can achieve the most delectable variations by using fresh, in-season produce: it can be a real joy to go to a market and select the vegetables that look most inviting. Furthermore, you can turn yourself into a gardener by growing a number of fresh herbs on your windowsill. Rosemary, thyme, basil, marjoram, chives, parsley, and more can be chosen to vary the taste of your soups and stews and simultaneously create a beautiful mixture of green in your kitchen—not to mention the olfactory joy they bring.

Dinner

Be "your guest" ... really treat yourself to a joyful, mindful meal in the evening. Remember that by the time the sun sets the brain has begun to receive messages to reduce the production of adrenaline, which is needed for proper digestion. So should you want to indulge in free-range meat, kindly do so well before sunset. Fish is usually digested in two hours, chicken takes a little longer, and red meat can take between four and six hours. Eating heavy meals late at night can make it difficult to sleep well. So should you come home late, why not create a lovely vegetable roast? Line your oven tray with foil, sprinkle with olive oil, and use a mixture of different root vegetables scattered with herbs. While your vegetables are roasting for about 30–40 minutes, it's the perfect time for your mindfulness meditation.

Mealtime tips
- Lay the table as if each meal was a special dinner date, for it truly is. How wonderful it is to have the gift of food in such abundance and variety. Light a candle and enjoy and really taste and smell every mouthful. Remember that gratitude is an important aspect of living mindfully.
- When you wash the dishes, feel the temperature of the water, the smell of the washing-up liquid, and the touch of the brush gliding over the surface of each individual dish. Thus a chore changes into a glorious opportunity to be mindful and grateful.

Case study: Miriam

In a routine health test Miriam had found out that her blood sugar was borderline diabetic. She hated the idea of having to take medication for the rest of her life. She also felt fearful when she found out the health risks that come with diabetes.

She decided to change her eating habits and eat with more awareness and joy.

First, she replaced her snacks, which had consisted of chocolate, cookies, and other high-sugar foods, with whole-wheat products and vegetable sticks. She then decided to invest a lot more time in planning and preparing meals that would release sugar slowly into her system. She also made sure that she never went for more than three hours without a little food, she increased her water intake and chewed every mouthful slowly.

In a short while Miriam, who was in her late forties, even learned to enjoy cooking. After a year her blood-sugar levels were stable, she did not need to go on medication, and she had lost over 25 lb in weight, which was a welcome side effect!

Guided Practice: Squash, Kale & Mixed Bean Soup

The soup in the first recipe here combines chunks of delicious squash with protein-rich beans and bright green, vitamin-rich kale. Its liquid stock and its vegetable content mean that the body will be refreshed by fluids, as well as food nutrients.

Vegetables can be the key ingredients of light meals, suitable for summertime or lunches on the go, but they can also be combined to create comforting, satisfying dishes. Sweet potatoes, butternut squash, and root vegetables, such as rutabaga or carrots, can be roasted or used in hearty stews and soups. Green vegetables provide a bitter and refreshing flavor contrast, and are packed full of iron and vitamin C, essential for a healthy body. Beans are cheap to buy, and provide a great, low-fat way of taking in protein and fiber, perfect for achieving and keeping the feeling of a full stomach, and healthy digestion.

Appreciate the changing aromas as the onion, garlic, and spices fry together when you begin cooking. Notice the subtle changes as you add ingredients. As the combined ingredients cook, notice that their juices blend with the stock to swell the soup, even as some liquid bubbles away in the cooking process.

Taste the soup carefully, testing the seasoning as you go. Check the texture of the vegetables—perhaps you prefer them with a bit of crunch. Let the soup cool gently before you begin to eat it. Use a wide, flat spoon, and sip the liquid slowly, taking care to chew the vegetables and paying attention to the way the soup's warmth affects how your body feels.

squash, kale & mixed bean soup

Calories per serving 182 • Serves 6
Preparation time 15 minutes • Cooking time 45 minutes

1 tablespoon **olive oil**
1 **onion**, finely chopped
2 **garlic cloves**, finely chopped
1 teaspoon **smoked paprika**
1 lb 2 oz **butternut squash**,
  halved, seeded, peeled, and
  diced
2 small **carrots**, peeled
  and diced
1 lb 2oz **tomatoes**, skinned
  (optional) and roughly
  chopped
13 oz can **mixed beans**, rinsed
  and drained
3½ cups hot **vegetable stock**
⅔ cup **half-fat crème fraîche**
3½ oz **kale**, torn into
  bite-size pieces
salt and **black pepper**

Heat the oil in a saucepan over medium-low heat, add the onion, and fry gently for 5 minutes. Stir in the garlic and smoked paprika and cook briefly, then add the squash, carrots, tomatoes, and mixed beans.

Pour in the stock, season with salt and black pepper, and bring to a boil, stirring frequently. Reduce the heat, cover, and simmer for 25 minutes or until the vegetables are cooked and tender.

Stir in the crème fraîche, then add the kale, pressing it just beneath the surface of the stock. Cover and cook for 5 minutes or until the kale has just wilted. Ladle into bowls and serve with warm garlic bread, if liked.

okra, pea & tomato curry

Calories per serving 176 • Serves 4
Preparation time 5 minutes • Cooking time about 20 minutes

1 tablespoon **groundnut oil**

6–8 **curry leaves**

2 teaspoons **black mustard seeds**

1 **onion**, finely diced

2 teaspoons **ground cumin**

1 teaspoon **ground coriander**

2 teaspoons **curry powder**

1 teaspoon **ground turmeric**

3 **garlic cloves**, finely chopped

1 lb 2 oz **okra**, cut diagonally into 1 inch pieces

1¾ cups **fresh** or **frozen peas**

2 ripe **plum tomatoes**, finely chopped

salt and **black pepper**

3 tablespoons grated **fresh coconut**, to serve

Heat the oil in a large nonstick wok or skillet over medium heat. Add the curry leaves, mustard seeds, and onion. Stir-fry for 3–4 minutes until fragrant and the onion is starting to soften, then add the cumin, ground coriander, curry powder, and turmeric. Stir-fry for another 1–2 minutes until fragrant.

Add the garlic and okra, and increase the heat to high. Cook, stirring, for 2–3 minutes, then add the peas and tomatoes. Season to taste, cover, and reduce the heat to low. Cook gently for 10–12 minutes, stirring occasionally, until the okra is just tender. Remove from the heat and sprinkle over the grated coconut just before serving.

AWARENESS POINTS

• Notice how the spices bring out the flavor of the vegetables. Use them in other vegetable dishes to bring them to life.

• Okra and coconut can be found in most supermarkets or grocery stores, but try to source unusual fruit and vegetables from local stores and markets.

• Freeze and keep this curry for a warming, but nutritional treat on a night in.

lentil moussaka

Calories per serving 304 • Serves 4 • Preparation time 10 minutes, plus standing • Cooking time 45 minutes

scant ⅔ cup **dried brown**
  or **green lentils**, rinsed
  and drained
13 oz can **chopped tomatoes**
2 **garlic cloves**, crushed
½ teaspoon **dried oregano**
pinch of **ground nutmeg**
⅔ cup **vegetable stock**
2–3 tablespoons **vegetable oil**
8 oz **eggplant**, sliced
1 **onion**, finely chopped

Cheese topping
1 **egg**
⅔ cup **soft cheese**
pinch of **ground nutmeg**
salt and **black pepper**

Put the lentils in a saucepan with the tomatoes, garlic, oregano, and nutmeg. Pour in the stock. Bring to a boil, then reduce the heat and simmer for 20 minutes until the lentils are tender but not mushy, topping up with extra stock as needed.

Meanwhile, heat the oil in a skillet and lightly fry the eggplant and onion until the onion is soft and the eggplant is golden on both sides.

Layer the eggplant mixture and lentil mixture alternately in an ovenproof dish.

Make the topping. In a bowl, beat together the egg, cheese, and nutmeg with a good dash of salt and pepper. Pour over the moussaka and cook in a preheated oven, 400°F, for 20–25 minutes. Remove from the oven and let stand for 5 minutes before serving with salad greens.

AWARENESS POINTS
- Notice the sounds of your cooking—the simmering and the sizzling skillet. Do you find these sounds relaxing?
- Are the colors of this dish ones you associate with healthy and nutritious food?
- Serve small portions, and eat slowly, noticing the signals from your body when you start to get full. Remember that while this is a vegetarian dish, lentils and eggs are filling foods.

fruity stuffed peppers

Calories per serving 421 • Serves 4
Preparation time 15 minutes • Cooking time 1 hour

2 **red bell peppers**, halved, cored, and seeded

2 **orange bell peppers**, halved, cored, and seeded

2 tablespoons **olive oil**, plus extra for brushing

1 **red onion**, chopped

1 **garlic clove**, crushed

1 small **red chile**, seeded and finely chopped

scant ¼ cup **pine nuts**

generous 1 cup cooked **wild rice**

13 oz can **green lentils**, rinsed and drained

8 oz **cherry tomatoes**, quartered

½ cup **ready-to-eat dried apricots**, chopped

handful of **golden raisins**

grated rind of 1 **lemon**

2 tablespoons chopped **fresh herbs**

¾ cup crumbled **feta cheese**

Put the bell peppers in an ovenproof dish, cut side up, and brush each with a little oil. Place in a preheated oven, 400°F, for 20 minutes.

Meanwhile, heat the oil in skillet, add the onion, garlic, and chile and fry for 2 minutes, then add the pine nuts and cook for another 2 minutes until golden. Stir in all the remaining ingredients.

Remove the peppers from the oven and spoon the stuffing mixture into the peppers. Cover with foil, return to the oven, and cook for 25 minutes, then remove the foil and cook for another 15 minutes. Serve with a crisp salad.

AWARENESS POINTS

- Apply the raisin exercise you learned on page 20 to a cherry tomato. When you slowly eat the tomato, notice the juice and the seeds. Is it sweet, or a little sour? How ripe is it?
- Do the same again with a piece of dried apricot and consider the ways in which it is different.
- What herbs did you choose? Take a moment, as you prepare them, to rub them in your fingers and to breathe their aroma.

greek vegetable casserole

Calories per serving 310 • Serves 4
Preparation time 10 minutes • Cooking time 25 minutes

4 tablespoons **olive oil**
1 **onion**, thinly sliced
3 **bell peppers** of mixed colors,
  cored, seeded, and sliced
  into rings
4 **garlic cloves**, crushed
4 **tomatoes**, chopped
7 oz **feta cheese**, cubed
1 teaspoon **dried oregano**
salt and **black pepper**
chopped **flat-leaf parsley**, to
  garnish

Heat 3 tablespoons of the oil in an ovenproof casserole or Dutch oven, add the onion, bell peppers, and garlic and cook until soft and starting to brown.

Add the tomatoes and cook for a few minutes until softened. Mix in the feta and oregano, season to taste with salt and black pepper, and drizzle with the remaining oil.

Cover and cook in a preheated oven, 400°F, for 15 minutes. Garnish with the parsley and serve with warmed crusty bread, if liked.

AWARENESS POINTS
- This recipe involves a riot of colors to enjoy—the beautiful, shiny bell peppers against the green herbs and the white feta, as well as crisped pepper skins and browned cheese.
- As your casserole warms, leave the room for a short while, and then as you come back in, appreciate the delicious smell of cooking.
- Perhaps you could increase the vitamin content by serving this with some dark green baby spinach leaves and sliced cucumber, with a drizzle of olive oil.

baked eggplants with tzatziki

Calories per serving 325 • Serves 4
Preparation time 10 minutes, plus cooling • Cooking time 50 minutes

2 large **eggplants**, halved
  lengthwise
1 tablespoon **olive oil**
½ cup **couscous**
¾ cup **boiling water**
1 **onion**, finely chopped
1 **garlic clove**, crushed
½ cup **ready-to-eat dried
  apricots**, chopped
scant ⅓ cup **raisins**
grated rind and juice of 1
  lemon
2 tablespoons chopped **mint**
2 tablespoons chopped **fresh
  cilantro**
2 tablespoons grated
  Parmesan cheese
4 **flat breads**, to serve

Tzatziki
½ **cucumber**, finely chopped
2 **scallions**, sliced
scant 1 cup **Greek yogurt**

Lay the eggplants cut side up on a baking sheet and brush each with a little of the oil. Cook in a preheated oven, 400°F, for 30–35 minutes until tender, then remove (leaving the oven on) and let cool. When the eggplants are cool enough to handle, scoop out the flesh and roughly chop. Set the skins aside.

Place the couscous in a heatproof container, pour on the measurement water, and cover with plastic wrap. Set aside for 5 minutes, then remove the plastic wrap and fork through.

Heat the remaining oil in a nonstick skillet, add the onion and garlic, and fry for 3 minutes. Stir through the apricots, raisins, lemon rind and juice, couscous, herbs, Parmesan, and eggplant flesh. Spoon this mixture into the eggplant skins and bake for 10 minutes.

Mix together the tzatziki ingredients in a serving bowl and serve with the eggplants and flat breads.

AWARENESS POINTS

• When cooking with a variety of fresh herbs, always take time to smell and compare them. Which of them do you find the most enticing?

• Notice how the eggplant skins overflow with the plentiful, nutritious filling. Think about how this warm, fresh food will nourish and sustain you.

• Take a moment to enjoy the different sensations in your mouth—the hot, grainy couscous, and the cool, creamy tzatziki. Do they work well together? Which do you prefer?

split pea & pepper patties

Calories per serving 312 • Serves 4
Preparation time 15 minutes, plus chilling
Cooking time 45–50 minutes

3 cups **vegetable stock**
3 **garlic cloves**
1¼ cups **yellow split peas**
olive oil spray
2 **red bell peppers**, halved,
    cored, and seeded
1 **yellow bell pepper**, halved,
    cored, and seeded
1 **red onion**, quartered
1 tablespoon chopped **mint**,
    plus extra leaves to garnish
2 tablespoons **capers**, drained
    and chopped
flour, for dusting
salt and **black pepper**

Tzatziki
½ **cucumber**, finely chopped
1 **garlic clove**, crushed
2 tablespoons chopped **mint**
1¼ cups **low-fat plain yogurt**

Bring the stock to a boil in a large saucepan. Peel and halve 1 of the garlic cloves, then add to the pan with the split peas and cook for 40 minutes until the split peas are tender. Season with salt and black pepper and let cool slightly.

Meanwhile, lightly spray a roasting pan with oil. Place the remaining garlic cloves in the pan with the bell peppers and onion and cook in a preheated oven, 400°F, for 20 minutes. Squeeze the roasted garlic cloves from their skins and chop with the roasted vegetables.

Mix together the split peas, roasted vegetables, mint, and capers in a large bowl. Shape into 12 patties using floured hands. Chill until ready to cook.

Make the tzatziki. Mix the ingredients together in a bowl, cover, and chill for 30 minutes before serving.

Heat a little oil in a skillet and cook the patties for 2 minutes on each side. Serve hot or cold, garnished with mint leaves and with the tzatziki.

AWARENESS POINTS
• When you work with the raw and the roasted garlic, how do the smells differ—has the aroma changed during the cooking process?
• How does the flour feel on your hands—is it a comfortable sensation?
• Beans are full of protein and fiber, and will fill you up. Notice how much (or how little) you need to eat before you are full.

caponata ratatouille

Calories per serving 90 • Serves 6
Preparation time 20 minutes • Cooking time 35 minutes

1½ lb **eggplants**
1 large **onion**
1 tablespoon **olive oil**
3 **celery sticks**, roughly
  chopped
a little **wine** (optional)
2 large **beefsteak tomatoes**,
  skinned and seeded
1 teaspoon chopped **thyme**
¼–½ teaspoon **cayenne pepper**
2 tablespoons **capers**
handful of **pitted green olives**
4 tablespoons **white wine
  vinegar**
1 tablespoon **sugar**
1–2 tablespoons **unsweetened
  cocoa** (optional)
black pepper

To garnish
toasted, chopped **almonds**
chopped **parsley**

Cut the eggplants and onion into
½ inch chunks.

Heat the oil in a nonstick skillet until very
hot, add the eggplant, and fry for about 15
minutes until very soft. Add a little boiling
water to prevent sticking if necessary.

Meanwhile, place the onion and celery
in a saucepan with a little water or wine.
Cook for 5 minutes until tender but
still firm.

Add the tomatoes, thyme, cayenne
pepper, and eggplant, and onions. Cook
for 15 minutes, stirring occasionally. Add
the capers, olives, wine vinegar, sugar,
and cocoa, if using, and cook
for 2–3 minutes.

Season with black pepper and serve
garnished with almonds and parsley.
Serve hot or cold as a side dish,
appetizer, or an entrée, with polenta and
hot crusty bread, if liked.

AWARENESS POINTS
- Notice the textures of the raw eggplants. What do you find appealing/off-
  putting about them?
- Eat a small piece of raw celery. What do you notice? Where in your head or
  mouth do you hear or feel the crunch? Do you like the taste?
- Did you choose to use unsweetened cocoa? How does it affect the flavor of the
  caponata? Is it sweet or bitter?

7 The simple things are the best—making food from scratch

When we entertain friends and family for a special occasion, we tend to put in extra time and effort and prepare food ourselves rather than buying ready-made. It becomes a ritual of sorts and can give us a heightened sense of wellbeing. It is well documented that gardeners and builders come top of lists of the happiest professions. Seeing something through from initial idea to completion, with plenty of tiny goals to achieve along the way, can be hugely satisfying. Now is the time to expand your thoughts about eating to include the wider community and the world. Where food comes from, and to whom it goes, is an essential part of mindful eating. The more we step back from the complex processes that food-production companies employ, the more we are able to appreciate that simple food can soothe the soul.

Making food from scratch, as discussed in this chapter, can be a rewarding pastime, as well as a reward when you sit down and eat it afterward!

Enjoy your bread

You may wonder what freshly baked bread has to do with mindful eating. Let me explain. By baking your own bread, even if you do it just once in a while, you will explore another aspect of what it means to live a mindful life. Making progress in practicing mindfulness by taking small steps encourages you to trust the process. Hopefully you have found some of the ideas and recipes in this book to be healing and nourishing, and to a certain extent, that is what can be said of making bread.

When we make our own bread, we engage in a process that seeks integrity. It requires time and patience, and reminds us that good things often unfold slowly, in their own time. It reminds us that less can be more—less noise in our head, more calm instead. This is so true in relation to bread.

Millions of loaves are sold in the US alone, but not all bread is as healthy as we are lead to believe. Store bread has been bleached, blanched, and stripped of its nutrients, which are then injected back into it. Most of the bread has high sugar and salt content, and various enzymes, preservatives, and additives have been included to extend its shelf life. It is highly processed, and we have been fooled if we think that this is real, authentic bread.

You might think that you don't have time to make your own bread, but please think again. By making your own bread, you will bring to mind some of the ingredients we need in our daily life, such as time and patience, authenticity, and simplicity. You will stay true to what is important—home, family, and friends, the wellbeing of others, and of the entire universe.

The time it takes for the dough to rise and ferment is important as it will neutralize the parts of the wheat protein that might trigger allergic reactions. Equally, we sometimes need to make time for ourselves to have a rest and to restore our energies. Sometimes we need time to go through difficult issues at work or at home, and it is better not to speed up the process, because that may result in fast but possibly unstable and unhealthy solutions.

As you bake your own bread, even if you do it occasionally, you are celebrating another mindfulness characteristic—simplicity; the ability to enjoy the simple pleasures of life—warm sun on the skin, the touch of a cat's soft fur, a hot dish on the table ready and waiting when you arrive home on a cold, wet evening. These are small pleasures but when we can bring mindfulness to them, we can experience a happiness we thought we had lost.

These simple pleasures are right in front of our eyes but so often we miss the opportunity to be touched by them because our mind is somewhere else. Somewhere along the way we have lost the ability to taste, hear, see, smell, and touch. Our desire always to have more of everything has lead to us losing our appreciation of the simple things in life.

Do you remember a time when you were really, really hungry? And when at long last you found a meal, wasn't that the best meal ever? When you are hungry, freshly baked bread with butter is the most amazing-tasting feast you can imagine. Sit, eat, and enjoy it. Complicated dishes are not necessary, just a mind that is able to feel the richness and deliciousness of the food in front of you. Don't read the newspaper or check your e-mails. Just enjoy the simple meal of bread and butter.

So now can you see how opening up to the present moment, to a simple meal, can bring you in touch with happiness? It is our spoiled mind that puts conditions on happiness. It thinks that only when things are perfect can we be happy. And what is perfect anyway? We so often miss the happiness that is right in front of us. Let go of this attitude, just for now. Enjoy the simple meal and experience the happiness it can bring you.

More ideas

It's not just baking bread that brings a happiness reward. Baking other food is a great way to spend an afternoon or weekend. From batches of scones to trays of cupcakes, you can chart the mindful journey it takes you on. Making jam is a great way to use home-grown fruit and to recycle jars (be sure to sterilize them first), and batch cooking can be great for busy professionals. Cook a hearty soup or stew that can be kept or frozen, so you can quickly heat up a healthy meal after work.

Guided Practice: A Very Happy Birthday Cake

One element of mindfulness is the idea of taking and giving back to the community. Mindful eating can be just as much about thoughtful gifts for others as it is about rewarding yourself. What can be more mindful than a homemade birthday cake? The thought of spending a morning or afternoon dedicated to celebrating somebody—or even yourself—is the ultimate gift. Watching very basic ingredients (flour, eggs, sugar) transform into something complex is part of the enjoyment. Then there is the smell of baking, licking the spoon, decorating the cake, positioning the candles—every attention to detail adds to the pleasure.

When you make the cake, enjoy the experience, wish kindness to yourself, and extend the thought of kindness to others. While the cake is baking, perhaps do a mindful exercise or body scan. Finally, make the cake as personal as possible.

Special touch

Here are some ideas for making a birthday cake really special with just some added thoughtfulness.

- Add a favorite ingredient to the sponge or filling.
- Spell out the recipients initials in strawberries.
- Buy a plate or cake stand to present it on as an added gift.
- Decorate a cake box with printouts of family photographs, your friend's favorite movie poster or your child's favorite TV character.

a very happy birthday cake

Calories per serving 430 • Cuts into 12
Preparation time 25 minutes, plus cooling
Cooking time 35–40 minutes

12 tablespoons (1½ sticks)
  slightly salted butter,
  softened, plus extra for
  greasing
generous ¾ cup superfine
  sugar
2 teaspoons vanilla extract
2½ cups self-rising flour
2 teaspoons baking powder
3 eggs
generous ¼ cup ground rice
⅔ cup low-fat plain yogurt

To finish
1¼ cups heavy cream
3 tablespoons reduced-sugar
  strawberry jam
1¼ cups strawberries, hulled
  and cut into wedges

Grease 2 x 8 inch sandwich pans and line the bottoms with nonstick baking parchment.

Put the butter, sugar, and vanilla extract in a food processor and blend until smooth. Sift in the flour and baking powder, add the eggs, ground rice, and yogurt and whizz together until creamy.

Divide the batter between the prepared cake pans and level the surface. Bake in a preheated oven, 350°F, for 35–40 minutes until risen, golden, and springy to the touch. Let cool in the pans for 10 minutes, then turn out onto a wire rack and peel off the lining paper. Let cool completely.

Whip the cream in a bowl until soft peaks form. Cut the top off one of the cakes to level it, then spread with the jam and then half of the cream to the edge. Scatter with two-thirds of the strawberries. Place the second cake on top and spread with the remaining cream. Scatter with the remaining strawberries or form them into the birthday girl or boy's initials. Add candles.

simple white loaf

Calories per serving 118 • Makes 1 large loaf
Preparation time 5 minutes
Cooking time 3–4 hours, depending on machine

generous 1 cup **water**
¼ stick **unsalted butter,**
  softened
1 teaspoon **salt**
3¾ cups **strong white bread**
  flour, plus extra for dusting
2 teaspoons **superfine sugar**
1¼ teaspoons **active-dry yeast**

Lift the bread pan out of the machine and fit the blade. Put the ingredients in the pan, following the order specified in the manual.

Fit the pan into the machine and close the lid. Set to a 1½ lb loaf size on the basic white program. Select your preferred crust setting.

Take the pan out of the machine at the end of the program and shake the bread out onto a wire rack. Dust the top with a little extra flour and let cool.

AWARENESS POINTS
• Using a bread machine is a quick and simple way to create a loaf from scratch. If you find having made a loaf of bread satisfying, why not progress to the mixed-seed loaf recipe, or even kneading the dough yourself?
• How does the yeasty smell of dough rising and bread baking make you feel? Does it make your kitchen seem like a different sort of place?
• Think about what would complement the fresh bread. Perhaps some homemade jam or salty butter. Notice the different tastes and textures as you eat.

mixed-seed bread

Calories per serving 129 • Makes 1 large loaf
Preparation time 5 minutes
Cooking time 3½–5 hours, depending on machine

1¼ cups **water**
¼ stick **unsalted butter**, softened
1½ teaspoons **salt**
3 tablespoons **sesame seeds**
3 tablespoons **sunflower seeds**
3 tablespoons **flaxseeds**
3¾ cups **malthouse flour**
1 tablespoon **brown sugar**
1¼ teaspoons **active-dry yeast**

To finish
milk, for brushing
extra **seeds**, for sprinkling (optional)

Lift the bread pan out of the machine and fit the blade. Put the dough ingredients in the pan, following the order specified in the manual.

Fit the pan into the machine and close the lid. Set to a 1½ lb loaf size on the wholemeal program. Select your preferred crust setting.

Just before baking begins brush the top of the dough with a little milk and sprinkle over some extra seeds, if liked. Close the lid gently.

At the end of the program lift the pan out of the machine, loosen the bread with a spatula if necessary, and shake it out onto a wire rack to cool.

AWARENESS POINTS
- Take a moment to try all of the seeds before you begin. Which do you like the best? What shape are they, and what color?
- Choose your crust setting, and decide whether you will sprinkle seeds on top. What texture do you want the outside of this loaf to have? What color do you want it to be?
- This recipe is for a nutritious, filling loaf. As you eat, notice when your body starts to signal that you are full, and find the right time to stop eating. You can always have more bread when you are hungry again.

chai tea bread

Calories per serving 302 • Cuts into 10
Preparation time 15 minutes, plus standing • Cooking time 1¼ hours

5 **chai tea bags**
1¼ cups **boiling water**
2 cups **self-rising flour**
1 teaspoon **baking powder**
1½ packed cups **light brown sugar**
10 oz **mixed dried fruit**
⅓ cup **Brazil nuts**, chopped
3½ tablespoons **butter**
1 **egg**, beaten

Grease a 2 lb or 2¼ pint loaf pan and line with a nonstick baking parchment.

Stir the tea bags into the measurement water in a pitcher and let stand for 10 minutes.

Mix together the flour, baking powder, sugar, dried fruit, and nuts in a bowl. Remove the tea bags from the water, pressing them against the side of the pitcher to squeeze out all the water.

Thinly slice the butter into the water and stir until melted. Let cool slightly. Add to the dry ingredients with the egg and mix together well.

Spoon the mixture into the prepared loaf pan and spread the mixture into the corners. Bake in a preheated oven, 325°F, for 1¼ hours or until risen, firm, and a skewer inserted into the center comes out clean.

Loosen the cake at the ends and transfer to a wire rack. Peel off the lining paper and let cool.

AWARENESS POINTS

- As the chai brews, breathe in the steam. Take one deep, slow breath, hold it in for a count of four, then slowly breathe out. Repeat a few times.
- As the tea bread bakes, can you smell the tea? Count how many different spices or smells you can identify.
- When you cut and eat a slice of the loaf, notice the difference between the moist inside and the crustier outside. Which do you prefer?

sweet carrot & rosemary scones

Calories per serving 236 • Makes 12
Preparation time 15 minutes • Cooking time 8–10 minutes

1¾ cups **stoneground spelt flour**, plus extra for dusting
2 teaspoons **baking powder**
½ teaspoon **cream of tartar**
2 teaspoons **rosemary**, finely chopped
2 tablespoons **superfine sugar**
3½ tablespoons **slightly salted butter**, chilled and diced, plus extra for greasing
scant 1 cup finely grated **carrots**
scant ½ cup **milk**, plus extra to glaze
marscapone and **jam or fruit jelly**, to serve

Sift the flour, baking powder, and cream of tartar into a bowl or food processor, tipping in the grains left in the strainer. Stir in the rosemary and sugar. Add the butter and rub in with the fingertips or process until the mixture resembles bread crumbs. Stir in the grated carrots and milk and mix or blend briefly to a soft dough, adding a dash more milk if the dough feels dry.

Knead the dough on a lightly floured counter until smooth, then roll out to ¾ inch thick. Cut out 22–24 circles using a 1¼ inch plain cookie cutter, rerolling the trimmings to make more. Place slightly apart on a greased baking sheet and brush with milk.

Bake in a preheated oven, 425°F, for 8–10 minutes until risen and pale golden. Transfer to a wire rack to cool.

Split the scones and serve spread with mascarpone and fruit jelly, if liked.

AWARENESS POINTS
- Keep back a piece of carrot when preparing the ingredients. Taste it carefully, noticing its sweetness. Smell the rosemary. Try to anticipate the flavor combination.
- How does it feel to rub the sugar and butter, and to roll and knead the dough? Is it satisfying? Notice the physical sensations in your hands.
- As you split the scones and spread with mascarpone and fruit jelly, mark the contrast in colors—the white of the marscapone against the bright fruit and golden scones.

tamarind & date chutney

Calories per serving 161 • Serves 4
Preparation time 10 minutes

7 oz **dried dates**, pitted and
  roughly chopped
1 tablespoon **tamarind paste**
1 teaspoon **ground cumin**
1 teaspoon **chili powder**
1 tablespoon **tomato ketchup**
scant 1 cup **water**
salt

Put all the ingredients into a food processor or blender and process until fairly smooth.

Transfer the mixture to a serving bowl, cover, and chill until required. The chutney will keep for up to 3 days in the refrigerator.

AWARENESS POINTS
• What sort of ketchup will you use in this recipe? An organic one might be healthier and more ethically produced, or you could even make your own.
• As you pit and chop the dates, notice their delicious stickiness and rich aroma. What will you serve the chutney with, to contrast with the dates?
• Think about how you could present your chutney. Do you have a small, decorative bowl, or a dish that is in some way special to you?

cherry & raspberry jam

**Makes 4–5 assorted jars • Preparation time 10 minutes, plus cooling
Cooking time 20–25 minutes**

2 x 15¼ oz packages **frozen
  pitted cherries**
2¾ cups **fresh raspberries**
2 lb **jam sugar with pectin**
1 tablespoon **butter**

Put the frozen cherries and the raspberries in a preserving pan. Cover and cook gently for 10 minutes, stirring occasionally, until the juices run and the fruit begins to soften.

Pour the sugar into the pan and heat gently, stirring from time to time, until dissolved. Bring to a boil, then boil rapidly until setting point is reached (5–10 minutes). Skim with a slotted spoon and stir in the butter.

Let cool for 10 minutes so that the cherries don't rise in the jars, then ladle into sterilized jars, filling to the very top. Cover with screw-top lids, or with waxed discs and cellophane tops secured with elastic bands. Label and let cool.

AWARENESS POINTS
- Taste the raspberries before you begin. Do the raisin exercise (see page 20)—put one small raspberry on your tongue and let it dissolve very slowly. Notice its tart sweetness and the texture of the seeds.
- Watch carefully as the jam reaches setting point and the consistency changes. Notice the process as the various ingredients become jam.
- How will you package your jam? Perhaps you could create some labels with special lettering.

summer vegetable soup

Calories per serving 248 • Serves 2
Preparation time 10 minutes • Cooking time 15 minutes

1 teaspoon **olive oil**
½ **leek**, cleaned, trimmed, and finely sliced
½ **large potato**, peeled and chopped
7 oz **mixed summer vegetables**, such as **peas, asparagus, fava beans,** and **zucchini**
1 tablespoon chopped **mint**
2 cups **vegetable stock**
1 tablespoon **crème fraîche**
salt (optional) and **black pepper**

Heat the oil in a medium saucepan, add the leek and potato, and fry for 2–3 minutes until softened.

Add the summer vegetables to the pan with the mint and stock and bring to a boil. Reduce the heat and simmer for 10 minutes.

Transfer the soup to a blender or food processor and process until smooth. Return to the pan with the crème fraîche and season with salt, if liked, and black pepper. Heat through and serve.

AWARENESS POINTS

• Rub a mint leaf between your fingers. What does the fresh smell make you think of?

• Before you cook them, look at your summer vegetables and notice the different shades of green.

• Taste the soup before and after you add the crème fraîche. Mark the difference it makes to the color and to how it feels on your tongue.

thai red chicken curry

Calories per serving 307 • Serves 4
Preparation time 15 minutes • Cooking time 40 minutes

1 tablespoon **sunflower oil**
3 **shallots**, finely chopped
3 **garlic cloves**, finely chopped
2 tablespoons **Thai red curry paste**
2 teaspoons **galangal paste**
14 oz can **reduced-fat coconut milk**
2 teaspoons **Thai fish sauce**
1 teaspoon **palm sugar** or **soft light brown sugar**
3 **kaffir lime leaves**
6 **boneless, skinless chicken thighs**, diced
handful of **Thai basil leaves** (optional)

Heat the oil in a saucepan over medium heat, add the shallots and garlic, and fry for 3–4 minutes until softened. Stir in the curry paste and galangal paste and cook for 1 minute. Mix in the coconut milk, fish sauce, sugar, and lime leaves and bring to a boil.

Stir in the chicken, then reduce the heat, cover, and simmer for 30 minutes, or until the chicken is cooked through, stirring occasionally. Stir in the basil leaves, if using, and serve.

AWARENESS POINTS
- Take the time to smell the ingredients before you start to cook with them. How do you find the pungent fish sauce and the spicy Thai basil smell?
- Do you know where your chicken came from? Is it free-range, or even organic? Think carefully about the source of your food when you shop.
- Serve your curry with brown rice for an extra-filling and fiber-rich meal.

home baked beans

Calories per serving 235 (not including toast) • Serves 4
Preparation time 10 minutes • Cooking time about 2 hours

2 x 13 oz cans **borlotti beans**,
  rinsed and drained
1 **garlic clove**, crushed
1 **onion**, finely chopped
2 cups **vegetable stock**
1¼ cups **strained tomatoes**
2 tablespoons **molasses** or
  light corn syrup
2 tablespoons **tomato paste**
2 tablespoons **soft dark brown
  sugar**
1 tablespoon **Dijon mustard**
1 tablespoon **red wine vinegar**
salt and **black pepper**

Put all the ingredients in an ovenproof casserole or Dutch oven with a little salt and black pepper. Cover and bring slowly to a boil.

Bake in a preheated oven, 325°F, for 1½ hours. Remove the lid and bake for another 30 minutes until the sauce is syrupy. Serve with hot buttered toast, if liked.

AWARENESS POINTS
- Beans are a great source of fiber and protein and a filling meal choice. Consider the taste, texture, shape, and color of borlotti beans. You could try this recipe with other kinds of beans, such as haricot or lima beans.
- Taste the sauce mindfully. How do these beans compare to store-bought baked beans? Are they more or less sweet, and are they as salty?
- If you are eating beans on toast, what do they make you think of? How do you feel?

8 Making connections

Most of us feel that something is missing from our lives and we tend to try to fill this emptiness with food.

At times, life feels as though it is a dull dish, without salt and spices. We are either waiting for something to happen to liven it up, or searching for the right combination of ingredients to lift us, so that life can feel exciting and bright. Tired of the same old routine, we nevertheless continue to get up, go to work, come home, watch TV, and go to bed, with just a few variations in between.

At other times, life feels as if it has never really begun. Everything appears mapped out, as sterile and tasteless as the plastic packaging that contains our ready-made food. We would like to try something new, but somehow it seems easier to stay put and complain about it ("better the devil you know ..."). Or we feel that life has bent and squeezed us. We are ready to rise and break free but are missing the support, inspiration, and direction to become what we feel we were meant to be—happy and living a meaningful existence.

Food has become another commodity in our lives that promises to give us everlasting happiness, or at least a taste of it. What we are searching for is nectar, a mythological symbol of the sweet happiness and satisfaction that we can taste if we turn back home to our true source.

Tips to brighten up your life
- Go somewhere different for lunch.
- Eat with a colleague you don't know well.
- Walk around the block before you have your meal.
- Organize a charity dinner.
- Try a different drink.
- Revisit the religion of your childhood.
- Go on a retreat.
- Try these new recipes; they're great for sharing!

If you ask yourself what you are really longing for and what it is that brings you true happiness, what would you answer? Many people say that they want to live together in peace, free from torture and war. They want to live in a world where there is enough for all to share, and to protect the beauty of the planet, so that future generations can continue to enjoy their lives. But when we look at the daily news another picture emerges. In some parts of the world, people are struggling with obesity and issues of too much food consumption while at the same time other people go hungry and don't even have clean drinking water. In our so-called civilized society, we have to face up to leaders who seem to care more about what is best for them rather than for the whole of society, and who live with greed, dishonesty, and corruption.

We can't change them, but we can make small changes in our own lives. We can remember our true longing, our true innermost being, and we can begin to nourish ourselves by appreciating what life has given us, and by sharing this with others. One way to do this is by eating together. How many families eat their meals separately? Eating with family and others can be your small commitment to living a meaningful and inspired life in which you acknowledge our shared human nature and interconnectedness.

Tips for shared eating

In a relaxed atmosphere with others, we often eat more than we really need. Here are some tips to help you avoid it.

• Start eating only when everyone else at the table has begun. This will help you to slow down from the outset.
• Listen more and talk less, so you can concentrate on eating slowly.
• Tune in with another person who eats slowly. Follow his or her speed. Enjoy more and eat less.

Sharing a meal with others can truly enrich your life. By cooking and eating together, even just for an evening, you can create a community that has values, such as not turning away strangers in need of food. Try taking it in turns to cook for one another, inviting new guests to share your meals, involving teenagers and encouraging them to join in and take turns.

Think of all the events that can happen around the table that are an expression of our shared lives. Here are some examples:

• Arguments and rows.
• Decisions big and small.
• Toasts, for example to newlyweds.

- Speeches at a funeral.
- Religious festivals.
- Sharing of recipes.
- Support during difficult times.

Food not only connects, though. We also have to be mindful of how food, and its production, can exclude others:
- Vegans and vegetarians are not always considered.
- Homeless people may go hungry.
- Migrant workers may be exploited.
- Food-processing plants often pay workers low wages.

The world's resources

Our journey toward mindful eating is slowly drawing to an end. It would, however, be incomplete if, as compassionate beings, we failed to consider the consequences of our eating habits and food production for the rest of the world. So let's think about what it actually means to eat, harvest, and sell food mindfully.

Our exploitation of natural resources and reliance on imbalanced food production have put our whole planet and its inhabitants in danger. In *Harvest for Hope: A Guide to Mindful Eating*, world-renowned anthropologist Jane Goodall writes about how easy it would be for all of us to improve the state of this earth if we became more aware of it and compassionate toward all beings. One reviewer of her book puts it in a nutshell: "Eat organic, locally grown foods whenever possible and you will be a healthier person and contribute to the health of our environment."

Everything is interrelated. For example, huge areas of the Amazon Forest are devoted to growing soy, which goes to feed cattle in Europe and Asia. These animals are the origin of the cheap meat we can buy from many supermarket chains. The animals have not been fed according to their needs, nor have the indigenous people had the opportunity and fair option to plant and grow the food they need for their own survival.

Another unbelievable fact is that 6,599 gallons of water are needed to rear 2 lb of beef. In many areas of the world, hardly anything grows at all because of a lack of water. Can we justify producing such huge amounts of meat?

Mindfulness in vegetarian and vegan food

Many people believe, rightly or wrongly, that eating less meat would improve their wellbeing. In Germany, a number of television shows focus on vegetarian or vegan cooking. Attila Hildmann not only inspires his nation but has been invited to America to demonstrate what he can cook without using meat, eggs, or milk products. Hildmann's first book, *Vegan for Fit*, challenges you to try his recipes for 30 days. Many of those who did claim that they have hardly ever eaten tastier or more delicious food.

In *Peace Food*, R Dahlke writes about the abominable treatment of animals in mass production. You need to be quite tough to read about how we make these animals suffer, and also to consider the harm caused to our environment and to the poorest of the poor. It is all interconnected. Shaun Monson's award-winning movie *Earthlings* is another source of information.

The sufferings animals have to go through are countless and severe. The way they are handled adds even more pain to the whole sad tale of mass meat production. It is hard to understand how human beings can be so unnecessarily cruel. Mahatma Gandhi is said to have commented, "You can gauge the greatness of a nation by how they treat their animals."

Mindfulness in organic food

One of the best-known studies on the connection between food consumption and health is the China-Cornell-Oxford-Project. Lead researcher T Colin Campbell points out how overconsumption of animal-based foods can lead to a number of degenerative diseases and early aging, to a large extent due to the lack of antioxidants. Hence more and more people choose to integrate larger proportions of fruit and vegetables into their daily diet.

Many indicators show that organic, and possibly even vegetarian, food improves overall health and can help you to maintain a healthy weight. In the end, each one of us has to decide whether to go for organically grown food and free-range products or not. They tend to taste better but due to smaller harvests cost more.

Maybe you could try asking yourself mindfully, "Can I really accept cheap products even though I know they may be responsible for the suffering of the poor, the animals and the soil of our land?" Even if 100 percent commitment to pain-free production of nourishment is not possible, it may still be preferable to apply some discernment whenever possible.

Conclusion

The food we eat and the food we buy matters. By being mindful, we build connections with others and make better choices. We understand what we really want. Mindfulness encourages us to enjoy the food in front of us, simple or rich, whether alone or with others, and reminds us that this is the first step. Try to go deeper and discover the inner nourishment of feeling your human connectedness and you will become less self-centered and more open. If you can achieve this, you will change your eating habits because you will know the impact you are having on others.

How to eat well without causing suffering to others

- Buy from local farmers.
- Use canvas bags for your shopping and refuse plastic ones.
- Eat produce that is in season and has not been flown from distant places. You will reduce your carbon footprint.
- If you must eat meat, choose organic and free-range.
- How about some mindful gardening? Grow your own herbs, fruit, and vegetables.
- Make your own jams and chutneys, from your homegrown products if possible—good for you and your family, and good as gifts for others (see pages 126 to 127). What a joy!

Food For Sharing Guided Practice: Baked Tortillas with Hummus

Whether going to a party or having friends over for a cup of coffee, an offering of light, healthy food is an important part of giving and receiving hospitality. The first recipe here makes a great snack for impromptu, casual gatherings, or a wonderful hors d'oeuvre for a more formal dinner party. It's perfect for vegetarians, full of flavor, and children will love the small hand-size pieces. It's very versatile, because you can simply offer raw vegetable sticks for a gluten-free alternative to the baked tortillas, or, if you prefer, swap the chickpeas for fava beans.

Tailor your creations to the people they are meant for, to show you have noticed their preferences. Homemade dips are quick to make, so you can spend extra time adjusting the seasoning and consistency. Does everyone like a lot of garlic? Perhaps you have a friend coming who would appreciate celery sticks, or a little less salt.

Notice how the smell of hot tortillas fresh from the oven brings a welcoming, warm feel to your home, and how good it feels to offer nutritious, comforting food to your friends. Allow extra time so that you can work on the visual element. You could achieve a lovely effect by displaying your dips in pretty bowls—or why not go for bohemian chic by using painted tin cups or jam jars? Perhaps you have a dish that one of your guests gave you—how would they feel if you made a point of using that? Finish your dips by topping with drizzled oil and a sprinkling of paprika, or add a fresh herb garnish. Arrange the baked tortilla triangles or crisp, colorful vegetables around them, creating a dazzling sensory experience for your guests.

baked tortillas with hummus

Calories per serving 312 • Serves 4
Preparation time 5 minutes • Cooking time 10–12 minutes

4 small **soft flour tortillas**
1 tablespoon **olive oil**

Hummus
13 oz can **chickpeas**, rinsed
and drained
1 **garlic clove**, chopped
4 tablespoons **Greek-style
yogurt**
2 tablespoons **lemon juice**
1 small bunch of **fresh
cilantro**, chopped
salt and **black pepper**
paprika, for sprinkling

Make the hummus first. Put the chickpeas in a bowl and mash with a fork to break them up. Add the garlic, yogurt, lemon juice, and cilantro and season with salt and pepper. Mix together. Alternatively, put all the ingredients, except the cilantro, in a blender or food processor and blend to a coarse puree. Add the cilantro and whiz briefly until mixed through. Put the hummus in a serving bowl or dish and sprinkle with a little paprika.

Cut each tortilla into 8 triangles, put on a baking sheet, and brush with a little oil. Bake in a preheated oven, 400°F, for 10–12 minutes until golden and crisp.

Serve the tortilla triangles with the hummus for dipping or spreading on top.

smoked salmon cones

Calories per serving 270 • Serves 4 • Preparation time 15 minutes

2 small **cucumbers**, halved lengthwise, seeded, and cut into thin strips
1 teaspoon prepared **English mustard**
1 tablespoon **white wine vinegar**
½ teaspoon **superfine sugar**
1 tablespoon finely chopped **dill weed**
2 **flour tortillas**
4 tablespoons **crème fraîche**
4½ oz **smoked salmon trimmings**, any larger pieces cut into wide strips
salt and **black pepper** (optional)

Put the cucumber strips in a shallow glass or ceramic bowl. In a small bowl, mix together the mustard, vinegar, sugar, and dill weed. Season well with salt and pepper, then pour over the cucumbers. Let stand for 5 minutes.

Cut the tortillas in half and lay on a board or counter. Spread 1 tablespoon crème fraîche over each tortilla half.

Divide the smoked salmon pieces between the tortillas and top with the cucumber mixture. Add a little salt and pepper, if liked, and roll up each tortilla to form a cone around the filling. Secure each cone with a toothpick, if liked.

AWARENESS POINTS
• These cones make wonderful finger food for sharing. As you prepare them, think who will be eating them, and consider the right size for holding and how tightly you should wrap them up.
• Notice the fresh smells of the dill weed and cucumber, and the sharpness of the vinegar and mustard.
• Take time to arrange the cones appetizingly on a platter, and make them attractive to your guests.

spanish fish stew

Calories per serving 328 • Serves 4
Preparation time 12 minutes • Cooking time about 25 minutes

2 tablespoons **olive oil**
1 large **red onion**, sliced
4 **garlic cloves**, chopped
1 teaspoon **smoked paprika**
pinch of **saffron threads**
11½ oz **monkfish fillet**, cut into chunks
8 oz **red mullet fillets**, cut into large chunks
3 tablespoons **Madeira**
1 cup **fish** or **vegetable stock**
2 tablespoons **tomato paste**
13 oz can **chopped tomatoes**
2 **bay leaves**
1½ lb **live mussels**, scrubbed and debearded (discard any that don't shut when tapped) or 8 oz **cooked shelled mussels**
salt and **black pepper**
3 tablespoons chopped **parsley**, to garnish

Heat the oil in a large, heavy-bottomed saucepan over medium-low heat, add the onion and garlic, and cook gently for 8–10 minutes or until softened.

Stir in the paprika and saffron and cook for another minute. Stir in the fish, then pour over the Madeira. Add the stock, tomato paste, tomatoes, and bay leaves and season with salt and pepper. Bring to a boil, then reduce the heat and simmer gently for 5 minutes.

Add the live mussels, cover, and cook over low heat for about 3 minutes or until they have opened. Discard any that remain closed.

Alternatively, if using cooked mussels, simmer the stew for 2–3 minutes more, or until the fish is cooked, then stir in the mussels. Cook for 30 seconds or until they are heated through and piping hot.

Ladle into bowls and garnish with the parsley. Serve immediately.

AWARENESS POINTS

• Pay attention to the sounds of cooking this dish, the sizzling of the onions, and the simmering of the sauce.
• How does the smell of the stew cooking make your kitchen feel? Do you have a bright tablecloth, or a set of red or yellow dishes you could use to make a cheerful and eye-catching presentation?
• What accompaniments would please the people who are sharing the stew? Think about what they prefer—salted or unsalted butter with their bread, or perhaps a dish of potatoes, or a dash of crème fraîche.

falafel pita pockets

Calories per serving 470 • Serves 4
Preparation time 15 minutes, plus overnight soaking
Cooking time 12 minutes

scant 1½ cups **dried chickpeas**
1 small **onion**, finely chopped
2 **garlic cloves**, crushed
½ bunch of **parsley**
½ bunch of **fresh cilantro**
2 teaspoons **ground coriander**
½ teaspoon **baking powder**
2 tablespoons **vegetable oil**
4 **wholemeal pita breads**
handful of **salad greens**
2 **tomatoes**, diced
4 tablespoons **fat-free Greek yogurt**
salt and **black pepper**

Put the chickpeas in a bowl, add cold water to cover by a generous 4 inches, and let soak overnight.

Drain the chickpeas, transfer to a food processor, and process until coarsely ground. Add the onion, garlic, fresh herbs, ground coriander, and baking powder. Season with salt and pepper and process until very smooth. Using wet hands, shape the mixture into 16 small patties.

Heat the oil in a large skillet over medium-high heat, add the patties, in batches, and fry for 3 minutes on each side or until golden and cooked through. Remove with a slotted spoon and drain on paper towels.

Split the pita breads and fill with the falafel, salad greens, and diced tomatoes. Add a spoonful of the yogurt to each and serve immediately.

AWARENESS POINTS
• Listen to the hard chickpeas rattle together when you first put them in to soak. See how that changes overnight as they become more moist.
• How does the mixture feel when you shape it into patties? Does it feel good to make something with your hands?
• Offer a feast of brightly colored salad options with the falafel pita pockets so the people you are sharing them with can choose their own vitamin-packed flavor boosts.

griddled vegetable platter

Calories per serving 285 (not including bread) • Serves 4
Preparation time 10 minutes, plus marinating
Cooking time 20 minutes

2 **zucchini**, sliced lengthwise into ¼ inch thick slices

1 **eggplant**, sliced lengthwise into ¼ inch thick slices

1 **yellow bell pepper**, cored, seeded, and cut into 1 inch thick slices

1 **red bell pepper**, cored, seeded, and cut into 1 inch thick slices

scant ½ cup **extra virgin olive oil**

2 **garlic cloves**, crushed

large pinch of **crushed dried red pepper flakes**

handful of small **mint** and/or **basil leaves**

salt

Toss all the prepared vegetables in 2 tablespoons of the oil until well coated.

Heat a ridged griddle pan over high heat until smoking hot. Add the zucchini and eggplant in batches and cook for 2–3 minutes on each side. Transfer to a bowl and toss with the remaining oil, the garlic, and crushed dried red pepper flakes. Set aside.

Add the bell peppers in batches to the reheated griddle pan and cook for 3–4 minutes on each side, then combine with the zucchini and eggplant. Season with salt and toss in the herbs.

Cover and let marinate at room temperature for 30 minutes. Serve with slices of country bread, if liked.

AWARENESS POINTS
- Enjoy the differing sounds and smells of sizzling vegetables—the freshness of zucchini against the sweet smell of bell peppers.
- How do the griddled veggies look to you? Do you find the darker lines across the flesh of the vegetables appetizing?
- Arrange the vegetables carefully on a serving platter, so that they look attractive and so that your guests are able to lift a nice selection easily onto their own plates.

beef & barley brö

Calories per serving 209 • Serves 6
Preparation time 20 minutes • Cooking time 2 hours

2 tablespoons **butter**
8 oz **braising beef**, fat trimmed away and meat cut into small cubes
1 large **onion**, finely chopped
7 oz **rutabaga**, diced
scant 1 cup diced **carrot**
½ cup **pearl barley**
8½ cups **beef stock**
2 teaspoons dry **English mustard** (optional)
salt and **black pepper**
chopped **parsley**, to garnish

Heat the butter in a large saucepan, add the beef and onion, and fry for 5 minutes, stirring, until the beef is browned and the onion just beginning to color.

Stir in the diced vegetables, pearl barley, stock, and mustard, if using. Season with salt and black pepper and bring to a boil. Cover and simmer for 1¾ hours, stirring occasionally until the meat and vegetables are very tender. Taste and adjust the seasoning if needed. Ladle the soup into bowls and sprinkle with a little chopped parsley.

AWARENESS POINTS
• Take a few moments to look at, and touch, the pearl barley before you begin. Where do you think the name originates?
• As this stew cooks very slowly, the smells become richer and deeper. When you uncover the pan to stir during cooking, take deep, slow breaths in and out, and enjoy the complex aroma.
• Notice the texture of the slow-cooked beef. Does it literally melt in your mouth or fall apart as you touch it?

lima bean & chorizo stew

Calories per serving 470 • Serves 4
Preparation time 10 minutes • Cooking time 20 minutes

1 tablespoon **olive oil**
1 large **onion**, chopped
2 **garlic cloves**, crushed
7 oz **chorizo sausage**, sliced
1 **green bell pepper**, cored,
  seeded, and chopped
1 **red bell pepper**, cored,
  seeded, and chopped
1 glass **red wine**
2 x 13 oz cans **lima beans**,
  rinsed and drained
13 oz can **cherry tomatoes**
1 tablespoon **tomato paste**
salt and **black pepper**
chopped **parsley**, to garnish

Heat the oil in an ovenproof casserole or Dutch oven, add the onion and garlic, and fry for 1–2 minutes. Stir in the chorizo and fry until beginning to brown. Add the bell peppers and fry for 3 minutes.

Pour in the wine and let bubble, then stir in the lima beans, tomatoes, and tomato paste and season well. Cover and simmer for 15 minutes. Ladle into shallow bowls, sprinkle with the parsley to garnish, and serve with crusty bread, if liked.

AWARENESS POINTS
- Mark the sounds of this dish as you begin to cook it—the sizzling onion and chorizo.
- When you add the wine to the hot pan, notice the strong, rich smell as it bubbles away.
- How will you serve the stew to your friends or family? Will you choose a wine they like, or bake them a special loaf of bread to go with it and serve it warm?

one-pot chicken

Calories per serving 275 • Serves 4
Preparation time 10 minutes • Cooking time 40–45 minutes

1 lb 2 oz **new potatoes**
4 **chicken breasts**, about
  4½ oz each
6 tablespoons **mixed herbs,**
  such as **parsley, chives,**
  chervil, and **mint**
1 **garlic clove,** crushed
6 tablespoons **half-fat crème**
  fraîche
8 **baby leeks**
2 **endive heads,** halved
  lengthwise
⅔ cup **chicken stock**
pepper

Place the potatoes in a saucepan of boiling water and cook for 12–15 minutes until tender. Drain, then cut into bite-size pieces.

Make a slit lengthwise down the side of each chicken breast to form a pocket, ensuring that you do not cut all the way through. Mix together the herbs, garlic, and crème fraîche, season well with pepper, then spoon a little into each chicken pocket.

Put the leeks, endive, and potatoes in an ovenproof dish. Pour over the stock, then lay the chicken breasts on top. Spoon over the remaining crème fraîche mixture, then bake in a preheated oven, 400°F, for 25–30 minutes until the chicken is cooked through and the vegetables are tender.

AWARENESS POINTS
- When you cut your herbs, take a moment to smell each one. Think about what each one makes you feel or remember. Which do you prefer?
- Think about how the food will look when it comes out of the dish, and spread the vegetables evenly.
- Eat this hearty, filling meal mindfully, remaining aware of the point where you are no longer hungry.

fennel & orange stew

Calories per serving 232 (not including polenta) • Serves 4
Preparation time 15 minutes • Cooking time about 50 minutes

2 **fennel bulbs**, trimmed
4 tablespoons **extra-virgin olive oil**
1 **onion**, chopped
2 **garlic cloves**, crushed
2 teaspoons **chopped rosemary**
3½ fl oz **Pernod**
13 oz **can chopped tomatoes**
¼ teaspoon **saffron threads**
2 strips of **orange rind**
2 tablespoons **chopped fennel fronds**
salt and **pepper**

Cut the fennel lengthways into ¼ inch thick slices. Heat half the oil in a dutch oven, add the fennel slices, in batches, and cook over a medium heat for 3–4 minutes on each side until golden. Remove with a slotted spoon.

Heat the remaining oil in the casserole, add the onion, garlic, rosemary, and salt and pepper and cook over a low heat, stirring often, for 5 minutes. Add the Pernod, let boil and boil until reduced by half. Add the tomatoes, saffron, and orange rind, and stir well. Arrange the fennel slices over the top.

Let the stew boil, then cover with a tight-fitting lid and bake in a preheated oven, 350°F, for 35 minutes until the fennel is tender. Stir in the fennel fronds, and serve the stew hot with some chargrilled polenta triangles, if liked.

AWARENESS POINTS
• Compare the taste of the fennel before and after cooking in stage one.
• Taste the sauce five times, focusing on, in turn, the garlic, rosemary, salt, Pernod, and orange.
• Does saffron have a taste? How would you describe it?

Mindful Food Production Guided Practice: Italian Broccoli & Egg Salad

There are some easy ways to ensure you know and approve of the source of your food. The first and most obvious is to grow your own. Why not start a windowsill herb garden, or grow a pot of rosemary outside? Tomatoes are easy to grow next to a south-facing window, and even the smallest garden or backyard has room for a mint bush.

Beyond exercising your green fingers, the next best way to be sure of where your food comes from is to buy locally. Even central urban areas have farmers' markets, and dates are advertised locally or online. Farm stores, neighbors who keep chickens, relatives with fruit trees—all these are good sources of absolutely fresh, organically produced food. Buy meat that has been organically reared, and make sustainable fish choices, including farmed trout.

Buying from smaller producers and retailers not only increases your chance of finding high-quality organic produce, free from the horrors of pesticides or unnecessary packaging, it also guarantees lower food mileage and supports local traders above faceless grocery store chains into the bargain.

The Italian Broccoli & Egg Salad given here is a great example of how mindfulness in choosing your food suppliers can improve the experience of eating. The yolks of farm-fresh eggs from uncaged hens are wonderfully yellow, and have a rich, delicious flavor. The organic, local vegetables will be fresher, sweeter, and better for you than those that have been sprayed with industrial pesticides.

Buy local, organic vegetables and, if possible, enjoy washing away the soil that they grew in, instead of discarding acres of slimy plastic wrap.

Boil your free-range eggs, feeling confident that the hens that produced them are leading healthy lives.

When you sit down to eat, savor the sweetness of the honey and the bite of the capers in the dressing, the soft eggs, and crunchy vegetable textures. Simultaneously, remember to appreciate the knowledge that, because you have bought locally produced vegetables and eggs, your meal is not costing the earth.

italian broccoli & egg salad

Calories per serving 211 • Serves 4
Preparation time 15 minutes • Cooking time 8 minutes

4 **eggs**
10 oz **broccoli**
2 small **leeks**, about 10 oz
  in total
tarragon sprigs, to garnish
  (optional)

Dressing
4 tablespoons **lemon juice**
2 tablespoons **olive oil**
2 teaspoons **clear honey**
1 tablespoon **capers**, rinsed
  and drained
2 tablespoons chopped
  tarragon
salt and **black pepper**

Half-fill the base of a steamer with water, add the eggs, and bring to a boil. Cover with the steamer top and simmer for 8 minutes or until hard-boiled.

Meanwhile, cut the broccoli into florets and thickly slice the stems. Trim, slit, and wash the leeks and cut them into thick slices. Add the broccoli to the top of the steamer and cook for 3 minutes, then add the leeks and cook for another 2 minutes until the vegetables are tender.

Make the dressing by mixing together the lemon juice, oil, honey, capers, and tarragon in a salad bowl. Season to taste with salt and pepper.

Crack the eggs, cool them quickly under cold running water, and remove the shells. Roughly chop the eggs.

Add the broccoli and leeks to the dressing, toss together, and add the chopped eggs. Garnish with sprigs of tarragon and serve warm with thickly sliced whole-wheat bread, if liked.

MORE RECIPES FOR MINDFUL FOOD PRODUCTION

zucchini, feta & mint salad

Calories per serving 169 • Serves 4
Preparation time 10 minutes • Cooking time 10 minutes

3 **green zucchini**
2 **yellow zucchini**
small bunch of **mint**
1½ oz **feta cheese**
salt and **pepper**

Dressing
2 tablespoons **olive oil, plus
  extra for drizzling**
grated rind and juice of 1
  lemon

Slice the zucchini thinly lengthwise into long ribbons. Drizzle with oil and season with salt and pepper. Heat a griddle pan to very hot and grill the zucchini in batches until marked by the griddle on both sides, then transfer to a large salad bowl.

Make the dressing by whisking together the oil and grated lemon rind and juice. Season to taste with salt and pepper.

Roughly chop the mint, reserving some leaves for the garnish. Carefully mix together the zucchini, mint, and dressing. Transfer to a large salad bowl, then crumble over the feta, garnish with the remaining mint leaves, and serve.

AWARENESS POINTS
• Zucchini and mint are very easy to grow yourself, if you have some garden or backyard space or even a large tub. Growing herbs is particularly low-effort, and you can freeze them if you end up with a larger harvest than you can use straightaway.
• Mark the contrasting flavors—the sharp, creamy cheese against the differently sharp lemon juice, and the freshness of the mint.
• Taste different flavor combinations with each slow mouthful.

roast vegetables & parsley pesto

Calories per serving 474 • Serves 4
Preparation time 15 minutes • Cooking time 50 minutes–1 hour

4 small **potatoes**, scrubbed
1 **red onion**
2 **carrots**
2 **parsnips**
8 **garlic cloves**, unpeeled
4 **thyme sprigs**
2 tablespoons **extra virgin olive oil**

Parsley pesto
½ cup **blanched almonds**
large bunch of **flat-leaf parsley**
2 **garlic cloves**, chopped
⅔ cup **extra virgin olive oil**
2 tablespoons grated **Parmesan cheese**
salt and **black pepper**

Cut the potatoes and onion into wedges and the carrots and parsnips into quarters. Put in a large roasting pan to fit in a single layer. Add the garlic cloves, thyme sprigs, oil, and salt and pepper and stir well until evenly coated. Roast in a preheated oven, 425°F, for 50 minutes–1 hour until browned and tender, stirring halfway through.

Make the pesto. Heat a heavy-bottomed skillet until hot, add the almonds, and dry-fry over medium heat, stirring, for 3–4 minutes until browned. Transfer to a bowl and let cool.

Put the almonds in a mortar or food processor, add the parsley, garlic, and salt and pepper and grind with a pestle or process to form a coarse paste. Transfer to a bowl, stir in the oil and Parmesan, and adjust the seasoning.

Serve the vegetables hot with the pesto.

AWARENESS POINTS
- If you have a large garden or backyard, growing your own vegetables is a great idea. If not, why not try parsley and thyme on your kitchen windowsill?
- Buying organic vegetables means more flavorsome, healthy food. Obtain organic ingredients for this recipe, and take the time to notice how different they taste compared with ordinary store vegetables.
- Take a moment to eat an almond before you begin, and mark its texture and taste. Notice how the almonds change in color and smell as you toast them, and try another when they are cooked. Which do you prefer?

trout with cucumber relish

Calories per serving 424 • Serves 4
Preparation time 10 minutes • Cooking time 10–12 minutes

4 **rainbow trout**, cleaned
1 tablespoon **sesame oil**
crushed **Szechuan pepper**,
 to taste
salt
chopped **chives**, to garnish
lemon wedges, to serve

Cucumber relish
1 **cucumber**, about 8 inches
 long
2 teaspoons **salt**
4 tablespoons **rice vinegar**
3 tablespoons **superfine sugar**
1 **red chile**, seeded and sliced
1¼ inch piece of **fresh ginger
 root**, peeled and grated
4 tablespoons **cold water**

Make the cucumber relish. Cut the cucumber in half lengthwise, scoop out and discard the seeds, and cut the flesh into ½ inch slices. Put in a glass or ceramic bowl. Put the salt, vinegar, sugar, chile, and ginger in a small bowl, then add the measurement water and mix well.

Pour over the cucumber, cover, and let marinate at room temperature while you cook the trout.

Brush the trout with the oil and season to taste with crushed Szechuan pepper and salt. Place the trout in a single layer on a broiler rack and cook under a preheated broiler for 5–6 minutes on each side or until cooked through. Let rest for a few moments, then garnish with chopped chives and serve with the cucumber relish and lemon wedges.

AWARENESS POINTS
• Think about the source of your trout before you shop for this recipe. Sustainable, farmed trout would be an ideal choice.
• If you can, grow herbs in your kitchen. Cutting your own chives is satisfying, cheap, and you can be sure of a lack of pesticides.
• Eat slowly and enjoy the subtle flavors of this simple, fresh dish.

The one-month mindful eating plan

This is an invitation to relearn the joy of eating well, so you can give up the completely unnecessary struggle to stick to a diet. Combine the one-month plan with the meal plan on pages 152–3, which gives suggestions for the first two weeks' meals. For weeks three and four, try to listen to your body's signals and choose your own recipes accordingly.

Week one:
—Do a mindful eating practice (see pages 20–22) on five separate days (or more if you like). Initially, it might be best to choose a short meal that you are eating on your own.
—In your journal (choose a fancy, funny, inspiring one) write down what you felt when eating mindfully. Ask yourself:
• Am I really hungry? How hungry am I—starving/fairly hungry/slightly hungry/not really hungry?
• Is my portion size appropriate for my hunger?
• Is it food I really want or other forms of nourishment e.g. relaxation?
—Practice one of the body scan exercises (see pages 16–18) on five separate days.
—At least five times during the week, engage in a mindful everyday informal practice, for example, a mindful shower, mindful brushing of teeth (see page 19).

Week two:
—Continue with the mindful eating practice (as in week one). Write down your feelings in your journal, as before.
—Try a mindful movement practice, such as mindful walking (see pages 62–3) or mindful swimming, on five separate days.
—Perform the body scan on two days.

Week three:
—Continue with the mindful eating practice (as in week one). Share a main meal with others (see Chapter 8 "Making connections") and try to eat half of it mindfully. Write down your feelings in your journal, as before.
—Do any of the breath awareness practices for 5–10 minutes (see pages 76–8).
—Do a mindful movement practice on five separate days.
—Perform the body scan on two days.

Week four:
—Continue with the mindful eating practice (as in week one). Focus on finding your triggers (see Chapter 5 "Destination guilt food"). Write down your feelings in your journal, as before.
—Do a mindful movement practice on five separate days.
—Alternate the body scan and the breath exercise—do one, once a day, five times during the week.
—Try something new (see Chapter 5 "Destination guilt food" and Chapter 8 "Making connections").
—Use your journal to write down anything you may want to remember for the future. Remember not to judge yourself—let go of the inner critic. Allow curiosity to be your guide.

And now ... do a selection from the above for the rest of your life.

Breakfast
Week one:
MON: Fig & honey pots
TUE: Layered nutty bars
WED: Oatmeal with prune compote
THUR: Green fruit salad
FRI: Mixed-seed bread
SAT: Frozen fruity yogurt
SUN: Poached eggs with spinach

Week two:
MON: Peach & blueberry crunch
TUE: Simple white loaf
WED: Fruity summer smoothie
THUR: Balsamic strawberries & mango
FRI: Citrus refresher
SAT: Chai tea bread
SUN: Home baked beans

Lunch
Week one:
MON: Warm chicken salad with anchovies
TUE: Zucchini, feta & mint salad
WED: White bean soup provençal
THUR: Spring minestrone
FRI: Smoked salmon cones
SAT: Roasted peppers with quinoa
SUN: Baked eggplants with tzatziki

Week two:
MON: Tomato & mozzarella salad
TUE: Miso chicken broth/Chicken noodle soup
WED: Squash, kale & mixed bean soup
THUR: Baked sweet potatoes
FRI: Butternut squash & ricotta frittata
SAT: Split pea & pepper patties
SUN: Falafel pita pockets

Dinner
Week one:
MON: Tuna steaks with wasabi dressing
TUE: Spiced beef & vegetable stew
WED: Chile & cilantro fish parcel
THUR: Sizzling Asian lamb burgers
FRI: Turkey râgout
SAT: Turkish lamb & spinach curry
SUN: Greek vegetable casserole

Week two:
MON: Salmon & bulghur wheat pilaf
TUE: Lima bean & chorizo stew
WED: Steamed citrus sea bass
THUR: Okra, pea & tomato curry
FRI: Lentil moussaka
SAT: Cashew chicken with peppers
SUN: Spanish fish stew

Mindful treats
Try to limit these to two per week:

Lemon & cardamom madeleines
Chocolate Florentines
Warm chocolate fromage frais
Passion fruit panna cotta
St. Clement's cheesecake
Toffee & chocolate popcorn
French macarons
Sweet carrot & rosemary scones

Index